Chris Donner
May 16, 2000

Confronting the Cow

A young family's struggle with breast cancer, loss, and rebuilding

---

by
C. B. Donner

CONFRONTING THE COW

Edited by
Mark D. Gustafson

Cover Design by
Ben Donner

Photo on back cover taken by
Bruce Unruh
(1996 Race for the Cure, Wichita KS)

ISBN 0-9679637-9-6
Library of Congress Catalog Card Number: 00-101674
Printed in the United States of America

Published by
Moonlight Publishing, LLC
4211 Peachway Drive
Durham, NC 27705
email : moonlightpublish@aol.com

*In
loving memory
of
Lisa Lusk Donner*

To *Karen, my wife and best friend, whose love and understanding made this possible.*

A special thanks to my children Samantha, Mackenzie, Emily, Ben and Gaven for constantly reminding me what is truly important.

Confronting the Cow

Foreword

Sometimes when I really need to relax I get a babysitter just so I can sneak off to the bookstore and hang out for a couple of hours. I get one of those large lattes with a sippy lid and walk up and down the aisles, occasionally dribbling coffee down my shirt while I run my fingers indiscriminately across the backs of the books. The smell is the best, the smell of all those new books. Maybe it's the glue or the ink, I'm not sure, but sometimes I pick up a book and flip through its pages real fast right in front of my nose. I might be an addict. I watch other people pretending to be reading as they flip through a book because I know that most of them are just book-sniffers like me. If they're actually reading, I try to guess what kind of person they are based on the book they've chosen. I know I would have a better shot at guessing their weight, but it's a form of recreation that doesn't cost anything.

On one occasion, however, I entered the bookstore and didn't notice the smell or even take time to get a latte. I was on a mission, actually looking for a book. I didn't know the title or the author. I wasn't even sure of the subject. It was one of those 'I will know it when I see it' deals, but I grew increasingly frustrated because I wasn't seeing it. After a while, I realized that it just did not exist. The book I was searching for was generally about men. Specifically, about a young man who has four small children and whose wife suffered a two-year battle with breast cancer and died. The young man was left on his own to raise his children, run a household, manage his career and resurrect a personal life. The book would talk about the changes this man went through as he endured each of the challenges that confronted him. The book I was searching for was about me, and it did not exist because I had not written it yet. I realized then that it was a needed book, and that it was my job to put that book up on the shelf so that others wearing similar shoes can find it.

This book is not another book about cancer, but it is a book written because of cancer and what it did to my family and me. This is not in any way going to be a clinical discussion. I will even refer to cancer as a 'cow' so that I have something dumb that I can get my hands on and punch. I am not an expert on anything. I am not an oncologist, radiologist, therapist, psychologist, sociologist, scientist, behaviorist or any other kind of 'ist.' I am just a guy whose family was eaten up and swallowed by a cow. The breast cancer cow. I have seen the cow from the inside so I feel in some way justified in having opinions about what life is like in there, but as I said, this is not

2

going to be about cancer. This is not even going to be about my wife, Lisa, even though she was the one the cow ate and kept. This is going to be a book primarily about my children and me and what we had to do to survive.

It is not possible to be eaten by the cow and not come out a different person. It is more than just a lingering stench that can be covered up cosmetically with sweet smelling colognes. It goes much deeper. I would even go as far to suggest that some of my chromosomes were altered, in some kind of sex change where the traditional bread winning, lawn mowing, male roles were mutated together with the mothering, shopping "female" roles. But it is much more than just the physical act of performing these female roles that I came to understand. I mean, just about any guy, including my untrained Father, can do some grocery shopping and laundry for a week and walk away saying, "What's the big fuss about?" The kids won't starve, they can wear socks that don't match, or even turn their underwear inside out for another day's wear. But if it's your full time responsibility day in and day out, then the seemingly little things become somewhat large and it does make a difference how they are done. It's feeling a daughter's disappointment when that favorite dress is wadded up in the dirty laundry and it is needed that day for a school performance. It's feeling a son's joy when the other kids in his class say "awesome" when you bring in a cool snack on snack day. These are the kinds of things that can make the difference between a good day and a bad day for children. If you can't feel what they feel then you probably won't do it right. If I could be so bold, I think this sort of behavior is more of a natural instinct for mothers than it is for fathers, and it's not a given that this trait can be acquired. Changes to these kinds of human or gender characteristics usually only come about as the result of a major life altering event such as a birth, illness, death or a Super Bowl. Even with that, it still requires that the capacity exist somewhere beneath the thick, tough layers of the stereotypical male skin.

My thick skin was constantly under attack by some very heavy artillery, which blasted holes big enough to drive armored tank-like changes through the surface. I can remember all too vividly when Lisa was in the hospital for five weeks for a procedure called a stem cell transplant. She had to stay in a special clean room that was free of germs, which meant that those walking germs disguised as our children were not allowed to see her. She was at such risk of infection that she was not even allowed to leave her room for almost four weeks. Not seeing her kids for a month had left her in a Mother's Hell. As soon as she was free to walk around the halls and visit the lounge of her prison, I drove the kids the 70 miles to the hospital so that they could stand outside the sidewalk and look up to the fourth floor lounge window. There they could see their mom. Her ghost white hands and forehead pressed against the glass shone like a beacon as she watched her babies jump and wave for what seemed to me (and the small crowd that gathered) like an eternity but in reality probably was all of five minutes. Then Lisa, whose strength was that of someone 100 years old, waved and went back to her room. The kids continued to look up for a moment longer as if waiting for an encore that they finally realized would never happen. Still smiling and chattering about finally seeing their mom, the kids and I got back in the car and drove the 70 miles back home.

What I had witnessed was this telepathic exchange of gut wrenching agony and unconditional joy between a mother, who was now only recognizable in her purest sense, and her children. At the time, I had no idea what deep-reaching effect this bombshell, and the many others like it, would have on my view of the world. I would find out later, but somehow Lisa knew how I was going to react. The knowledge that I would take good care of the kids and that they would somehow be okay is what allowed her some peace of mind.

I never would have imagined the compassion I developed for my kids as every move I made was directed toward their care. I began to develop that sense of a mother's love for her children, something I really could not have understood before. I became obsessed with doing laundry and cleaning floors, as if I had to prove that I could do these things by myself. I received a great deal of satisfaction from going to the schools for conferences with the kids' teachers, who commended me for the job I was doing. I began to develop that sense of what it really feels like to take care of children completely. From wiping their bottoms to putting that special snack in their lunch, and making sure that their favorite shirts are clean for picture day. It became all consuming, and my mindset shifted so that every decision I made had to go through a kid checklist.

I had absolutely no idea what mothers go through day in and day out. There were so many things that I had taken for granted, like getting a babysitter. I had no appreciation for how involved this could be and how important it was to be connected in the cult-like 'mommy network.' The deals that went down in grocery store parking lots or at the bus stop were totally unknown to me. Swapping a babysitter for a carpool pickup was not uncommon. Stealing someone's babysitter was grounds for being banished from the network. Casual conversation between two women at the store was really a network rendezvous. If I was going to survive, I had to get into the 'mommy network,' a place where men usually were not allowed. But, because of my situation I was given an honorary membership. It did not come with instructions so I had to figure out the rules as I went, being careful not to commit any major violations. I was now a man who was forced to live in a predominantly woman's world, while necessarily keeping at least one foot in the "man's" world.

Prior to the cow's arrival, my family was this young, green, sweet smelling, clover patch dominated by four kids. The oldest was six and the youngest was in diapers. Lisa and I both were 35 years old and we were on cruise control. I had a steady job and Lisa stayed home with the kids in our four bedroom, two-car garage house in suburbia. Then one day without warning the cancer cow came grazing indiscriminately through our lives. The cow has no feelings. It does not care if you are young or old, rich or poor, good or bad. It is just a dumb animal with the need to feed. The way I see it we were at the wrong place at the wrong time, and the damn cow ate us. It chewed on us like cud and we prayed that it would spit us back out before too much damage was done, but that was not the case.

Two years later I passed completely through the cow and squeezed out the other end, right beneath an uplifted tail. Plop. I stood and tried to see through all the crap covering my eyes and move my feet as I waded through the pile of manure produced by this cancer cow. I found my kids lying in a pool of sour milk. Its smell may not linger on them as long as that which permeated my body, but for now its foul, school cafeteria stench was nauseating. We all stood stunned for a moment as we tried to figure out what had happened to us, looking around for a mom that we knew was gone. My kids looked at me like that little bird who had fallen out of his nest in the children's book 'Are You My Mother?' I said "No, but I will do the best I can."

As the cow moved on, I wanted to let it go and put it somewhere in my mind where I could never find it again, but it is not that easy. I reached up and grabbed onto its tail. I could not just let it walk away from me after what it had done. It swung me back and forth swatting other flies like myself. I hung on.

I had a good friend who had been eaten by the same cow. She was young, scared and had no clue how to do this cow thing. I wasn't sure what I could do, but she seemed comforted by the fact that I had been through it, could understand what was happening and might have some thoughts about what may lay ahead. Her battle with cancer lasted for a year past Lisa's and I was exposed to many of the same horrors again, only this time it was being done to someone else's family. I helped her willingly because I knew that on some level I was making a difference. She asked me questions about how and why Lisa and I had done the things the way we had. She grilled me for hours like a witness to a murder. She needed to know the details of the thought processes we went through when making decisions regarding treatments, hiring hospice services, enduring the actual event of Lisa's death, and planning the funeral. My friend had young children as well, and her questions always were understandably slanted toward the effect our actions had on our kids. She used me for a sounding board. She wanted to know how my relationship with Lisa changed during the illness. She had so many questions, and as I stumbled over my answers I could see how she latched onto every word as if I were the ancient sage of truth sitting on top of this mountain of cow shit. She had traveled a long, hard road to get to me and did not want to miss a single word, or waste a precious moment because she did not know how many moments she had left. It frightened me to think that the words that came out of my mouth might truly impact decisions regarding the life of someone other than my kids or me. I can only imagine the pressure physicians must feel in dealing with this every day. The good ones are underpaid.

She took what I said and packed it away with all the other pieces of string, bottle caps, wire, and duct tape that she had gathered from under couch cushions, and from behind the refrigerator. I could see her sitting in a small room at a drafting table where she dumped out everything from her bags and pockets and was piecing together a plan for what remained of her life. What I had told her was not 'the truth,' it was simply my story, but hopefully it served as glue that helped to hold her plan together and allowed her to carry it out with greater confidence.

What she did for me was force me to go back and really look at what was going on in my head while I was engulfed by the cow. I realized that most of what I was doing was reacting, following gut instincts. There was not a neatly laid out plan for what we were going to do and how we were going to do it. In a way it was like wearing a blindfold in a boxing match with 'Rocky' and being forced to wait until he hit us with a punch so that we could feel where it was coming from and then try to throw a counter punch. We just wanted to go the distance.

It was amazing to me now, even with all the superhuman help and support we received from family and friends, that my kids and I came out of this, without the aid of straight jackets and stretchers. I still wish that someone who had been through the cow from my perspective had been available to talk things over with me. Not so much to give me the answers (although answers would be a plus), but at least to help me determine if I was even in the ballpark. I spoke with everyone who would listen, preachers, parents, brothers, in-laws, friends, and even the old guy at the end of the street who wore the same pair of pants every day. I looked for books to read, searching for anything that could give me some guidance. Everyone had well-meaning advice and the books had some good general information intended for a wide audience. But no source could get down to 'my' laundry level.

After my friend died I very passionately thought that I needed to stay close to this cow, as if it was what I had been put on this earth to do. I started doing volunteer work and speaking to support groups. I would drag my kids to support groups because I thought that they needed to keep talking about their mom and getting their feelings out. Every time one of my kids displayed some angry or sad behavior I would cock my head and try to determine if it was related to their mom's dying. Then, trying to sound like some junior 'ist' of some kind, I would ask them something dumb like "Are you mad at your mom for dying?" Family and friends kept asking me if the kids were seeing any special 'ists' because you never can tell what's going on inside their heads and so on. I started to get paranoid, and stopped doing what had worked so well in the first place. I needed to listen to, talk to and watch my kids. They had always been my measuring stick when I really took the time to notice what was going on with them.

Children, well at least mine, can't help expressing themselves by their actions. They don't have to verbalize much because it is written all over them. Sometimes they did actually write it out for me. A few days after the funeral, my son started his 4 year-old preschool class, and as is the case in preschools everywhere the first week is always "family week." The teachers asked Ben to draw a picture of his family. He drew the faces of all the people in his family, including his mother, and proceeded to fill the rest of the sheet with other unknown faces. He then went through with his marker and scribbled over all of these non-family faces. "Ben, who are all these people that you marked out on your picture?" asked his teacher.

"They are just people," he answered quietly.

"Are they bad or mean people? Why did you cross them out?"

Ben thought for a second and then said, "No, they are not bad people. They are all very nice, but I just want them all to stop looking at me."

When his teacher showed me the picture and told me of Ben's explanation, it made perfect sense to me. All of these people had been going through the revolving front door of our house. There were also all of the people who had come to the funeral. There were great aunts, great uncles, friends from work, and people from church. All of these people were patting him on the head, giving him hugs, telling him how sorry they were. The fuss that these unknown people were making, al-

12

though well intentioned, had been more than enough for Ben. All he wanted was to be a normal kid. He wanted the cow to go away so that he could play.

It seems to me that maybe the younger they are, the sooner they need to distance themselves from the cow. At least enough so that they don't feel like freaks in a side show where everyone is pointing and whispering. This is my unofficial opinion and is, of course, something for the 'ist' people to decide on.

This all sank in for me when I was taking them to a Saturday morning support group for children who had lost a parent. They went in bouncing and smiling and came out slumping and scowling. They never said much, other than that they didn't like it and didn't want to go anymore, which sounded like something they said when I asked them to go take a bath. There was something deeper there that I could see in the way their faces were twisted and in the tenseness of their bodies. It was then that I realized that it was time to give the cow a push. I was shoving this stuff down their throats but they were already so full that they were choking on it and needed a little bit of time to digest. In no way am I suggesting that kids who go through an experience like losing their mom don't need professional help, because I am almost certain that at some point they all do. I was told and had read that grieving comes and goes in waves or cycles, and from experience I can say that those "ist" people are right on that point. Once I understood this phenomenon it became easier for me to deal with my kids when they started bouncing off the walls. I began to expect it and looked for signs that something new was going on. All I am trying to do is to stay close enough to feel those waves as they come rolling in, and to determine whether my kids need that extra help or just some time and space to work things out on their own.

Consciously letting go of the cow was a big step for me, as it allowed me to start moving forward and really living again. I was re-energized, and started putting more effort into my career and social life. I took the opportunity to wipe the slate clean and do some things that I had always wanted to do, like playing ice hockey and writing. As I let go, that bone-wearying burden of hanging on was gone, and I felt years younger and stronger than I could remember. My kids, whom I had kept in my back pocket, needed me to get to this point. They too were free to feel good about themselves without always being reminded that they did not have a mother. As they flourished, the sympathetic head pats and hugs went away and a sense of normalcy settled in at our house. There are those who might view my actions and sentiments as being in some way disrespectful to the memory of Lisa, but nothing could be further from the truth. Each of us in our family thinks of her every

14

single day. But there is a fine line between holding on to memories and letting go of the cow. For so long that line was blurred, but as we detach from the cow, the kids' memories of their mother become more pleasant, which is just the way it should be.

Just because I let go of the cow does not mean for a second that I have forgotten that it is out there. I cross paths with it all the time. I read about it in the paper, hear it being discussed at work, and sometimes I go out in search of it for a specific reason such as participating in the 'Race For The Cure,' which is a fundraising event for breast cancer research. I know the cow will be present there. I go out of respect and love for Lisa, and in support of those people who don't have the choice to let go.

The tricky thing about cancer cows is that sometimes you can't always tell where they are. You could be standing in an elevator with a person, or be next to someone in the grocery store checkout line, that has been eaten by a cow. When Lisa was near death, delirious on morphine and breathing the manufactured air of the 24-hour a day oxygen machine, I would look out the window at cars passing by and think "The people in those cars have no idea of the pain in this house." It made me wonder as I drove through the neighborhood what other unknown atrocities were going on, what kinds of cows were living next door. I think twice these days before judging people.

Now as I come to my senses I am once again off in search of cows. I was given an overdose of reality and it almost killed me. I wish I could have taken this experience in small doses, like a daily vitamin. There is no doubt that I have come out of this a different, more complete, and more awake person. Unfortunately, that growth came at the expense of the life of a devoted wife and beloved mother. I can't change that, nor can I bottle up the lessons in cartoon-shaped reality vitamins so others can get my recommended daily allowance. But if I can put my experience down on paper to share with others, perhaps it will help someone who is dealing with similar realities or help someone appreciate what a loved one is going through. I hope it does.

Fat, Dumb and Happy

It was 5:30 on a typical Sunday morning. Like a shadow I slid silently across the kitchen floor in my stocking feet carrying my shoes in one hand and my red cooler in the other. It would be a cold dog day in Alabama before I would get to play golf again if I were to wake any of the babies before their time.

I had taken every precaution to ensure that my pre-golf preparation was accomplished as quietly as possible. Everything from going into the laundry room to load the ice in the cooler, to disengaging the automatic garage door opener so it could be lifted by hand without using the noisy motor. I put the car in neutral and pushed it out of the garage and to the end of our long driveway so that when I started the engine it would be as far from the house as possible. So far, so good.

As I loaded my clubs and cooler into the Jeep I couldn't help getting a bit excited. I loved that car. But, as always, the moment was tainted by the unavoidable flashback of Lisa crying on the day I traded in my motorcycle and drove home in the Jeep. One

17

of my friends was with me and I thought that I was Mr. Cool when I parked it in my garage. I was showing my buddy all the space in the back for clubs and coolers when Lisa entered the garage, took one look at the car, and started bawling. "What's the matter? You knew that I was thinking about buying this car."

"Yeah but I never thought you were actually going to do it," she said fighting back the tears.

"It's plenty big. There is room for two car seats, and by the time the baby is born Samantha won't need one. So I don't get what the problem is," I said defensively.

"Of course you don't get it. This thing is only a two-door," Lisa said frostily as the irritation started to overcome the tears.

"The front seat pushes forward and you just crawl in," I countered while demonstrating.

"I would like to see you try that when you're eight months pregnant and have to pull a thirty pound child out of her car seat. But I am so glad that there's plenty of room for your clubs and coolers of beer," Lisa said in disgust as she headed back into the house.

"It's still a ton better than my motorcycle," I shouted as the door swung shut. Then I looked at my buddy and said, "Man, I just can't win."

My inconsiderate choice of vehicles eventually would

catch up to me. A couple of years later I would be seen driving the Jeep to a car dealership and driving home in a plum colored mini-van with a sliding side door that was big enough to drive a golf cart through. For me this was truly the nightmare car from hell. In two short years I would go from driving a motorcycle, to a Jeep, and finally to a mini-van. Fortunately, at the time I sold my motorcycle I did not know that a mini-van was in my not so distant future and was therefore content because I had my Jeep.

The day's first rays of sun struck my face and the sound wave of mooing cows snapped me out of my flashback funk. I lowered the garage door and quickly poked my head into the house to listen one last time for the sounds of crying babies or the patter of little feet. "Look who's awake Daddy, it's Emily, and she really wants to see you," Lisa said as she handed Emily to me. "Judging by the smell I would say that her diaper needs changing. Maybe if you give her a bottle she would even go back to sleep, which is where I am going," she said as she headed back toward the bedroom.

"I'm supposed to be at Vin's apartment in fifteen minutes," I pleaded.

"Have the boys break their Sunday morning communion service and drink their Bloody Mary's in the car," she retorted from around the corner.

Quickly I got Emily a bottle and changed her diaper.

"Girl, what are you smiling about, you had better go back to sleep real fast," I said trying not to breathe through my nose. I would never get used to that smell. Then I put her in a little baby cradle with a handle and I swung her back and forth while she sucked on a bottle of that disgusting formula. Luckily for me, she fell back asleep. I placed her gently back in her crib and snuck out the door.

On this Sunday, play was unusually slow and by the time we finished 18 holes, had a beer and made it back home it had been at least eight hours. We took a few extra minutes to stop along a country road to see who could hit a golf ball closest to one of the cows grazing out in the nearby field. Lisa (who was five months pregnant with Ben) and the two girls were outside in the front yard when I pulled into our driveway. It was one of those hot, sticky (diaper) days in Alabama, where it was too warm for the kids to wear anything but a diaper. The wading pool was filled up and Lisa was kicking at our dog, trying to keep its big, slobbery tongue out of the water. As I stepped out of the car, I was greeted by two very wet hugs, a long wet tongue, and one cold shoulder. The long wet tongue belonged to my dog.

"How much money did you lose," she said sharply, as she snatched the keys out of my hand. "I'm going to the store. Why don't you try to have some fun with your kids and don't let anyone drown while you're mowing your lawn."

At this point, any kind of response would only have made

matters worse, so being the smart guy that I was I stood there with a stupid look on my face and said nothing.

As soon as she drove out of sight the dog jumped in the pool and started lapping up water. As predicted, I pulled the lawn mower out of the garage, put Emily on my back in a backpack, and proceeded to cut the grass with Samantha trailing behind me with her play mower.

I don't mean to make Lisa sound like a hen-pecking nag, because she wasn't. The truth was that she worked harder all week taking care of the kids and the house than I did snoring through meetings all day. She had a right to be more than a little bit perturbed when I consistently exercised my manly right to spend my day off playing golf.

What was it about golf that made me sneak around in my socks before the crack of dawn and leave my family on my day off? What made mowing the grass more important than spending some time splashing in the kiddy pool with my diaper-clad children? Where did my priorities and values (or lack of same) come from?

I had rehearsed in my head many of the rationalizations that all made perfect sense to me, but none of them ever sounded very convincing when I was defending myself to Lisa. It always came out sounding like I, I, I and me, me, me. She always came back with us, us, us and we, we, we. Still, I walked away grumbling, needing to play golf. There are probably reams of textbook material written by an "ist" person that attempt to explain this phenomenon. I have my own theories that justify my behavior completely, but I can only speak for myself and wonder if I have anything in common with the general golfing, lawn mowing male populace.

My strong need to play golf could have been based on my prowess at the sport, if not for the fact that I kind of suck. Or maybe I needed to play simply because I enjoyed it so much. But if you were to hear the Sunday morning prayers that came so frequently out of my mouth after an errant shot ("God, I hate this f@#%ing game!") you could make a strong case to the contrary.

Maybe it was the camaraderie that made golf so appealing and necessary. Guys need to hang out with "the guys." The group I played with was pretty fun even though I didn't have that much in common with them. They were all better golfers than me, but they were also either single or divorced and had no kids that they were aware of. Maybe there is a connection between being a better golfer and being divorced. But I would never trade my situation for theirs, especially in the name of golf.

After discounting all the obvious choices, the only rational theory that I can come up with for what drives me to do stupid things to play golf is one that blames it all on my distant relative, the Neanderthal Man. This hairy-backed creature (who I am rapidly beginning to resemble) most likely got together with other grunts-men in the early morn, leaving his family and the comfort of his cave with club in hand. Then he and his compatriots spent the day roaming the countryside making obscene noises and looking for things to hit with their long sticks. At the end of the day they would come home, squat around the fire and revisit every swing of their club while the women brought them food. There, that's my theory. It's in my blood, and to deny myself this instinctive activity would be like caging a wild animal and would promote sulky, self-pitying, depressive behavior. Take my advice and don't try to use this theory on your wife. It doesn't fly very far.

Lisa was due to give birth to our fourth and final child, a girl named Gaven (which has turned out to be the opposite of a boy named Sue), in the spring of 1993. We would then have our full complement of three girls and one boy, with four years and eight months separating the oldest from the youngest. For what seemed like forever, our house had been decorated in contemporary diaper with an aromatic mixture of baby wipes and baby poop. When we finally figured out what caused babies, we decided to make sure that it didn't happen again. Lisa suggested this thing called 'abstinence.' I looked it up in the dictionary and came to the conclusion that this form of birth control only works when you are not having sex. The other type of birth control that was being strongly suggested was a vasectomy. I was told that it would work whether we had sex or not and it was a much easier procedure than what women went through to achieve the same result. I could not deny that by giving birth to three (and soon to be four) babies Lisa had sacrificed her body enough for a lifetime. So, to prove what a good guy I was, I said okay to the big "V" and my new salutation included the display of two fingers. In the 60's those two fingers stood for peace, in the 90's (at least for Lisa and I) it stood for peace of mind. After it was too late to change my mind I realized I should have looked "vasectomy" up in the dictionary before I had agreed to go through with the procedure.

My operation was scheduled to be performed when Lisa was still four months pregnant with Gaven. The doctor said that normally they recommend delaying the procedure until after the last baby is born, just in case something were to happen to the child and the couple would want to try again. But when he found out that we already had three kids and saw the look on our faces, he knew that regardless of what happened we were done getting pregnant.

I then had an opportunity to find out what it was like for women to have their feet up in stirrups. First this young nurse invited me to this back room for a strategic shave and sponge bath. The next thing I knew, I was lying on my back, with my feet spread wide in those stirrups, wearing nothing but a white sheet, which was loosely draped across my legs. When that nurse opened a drawer and pulled out a new 5-pack of Bic razors she started to look more like "Edward Scissor Hands" and I began to feel a bit vulnerable. After receiving the closest shave of my life, the doctor walked in and gave me some well-placed shots of novocaine. He waited almost long enough for the novocaine to take affect and then made a couple of tiny incisions. I was still feeling pretty much intact until I saw the thin lines of smoke twisting and spiraling slowly up to the air vent in the ceiling directly above my crotch. In my mind I pictured the doctor with a soldering gun or arc welder, like the one I used in junior high shop class. At this point I realized that the next time my loins fathered another child it would have to be an act of God. The best part of this operation was that I was told I had to stay off my feet for three days and take plenty of pain pills. Of course every time I tried to lay down one of my loving children would come and jump right on my crotch. Why do they do that?

After just one day of staying off my feet I got bored, so I took a couple pain pills and mowed the lawn. I paid for this macho-mistake a couple of days later as I swelled in areas that were not meant to be iced down.

Lisa had worked until our second child was born, after which she could no longer bear to think of her babies being taken care of by some sweet old lady at a church while she sat and crunched numbers on a computer for some gigantic company. To us it was well worth the loss of her income for Lisa to stay home and take care of our children. It was one of the happiest moments

25

of her life when she sent in her letter of resignation in the name of motherhood.

Lisa and I had worked for the same gigantic company, which is where we first met. My job was very secure, paid better than average and had a great benefits package, which included a superior retirement plan that (if I could stick it out) guaranteed I would retire a millionaire. The stress level was low, as the pace of my job was similar to the Alabama lifestyle, slow as paint. It was an easy place to go every day.

There we were, fat, dumb and happy. Lisa was doing exactly what she wanted to be doing, which was staying at home and being a mom. I had this steady job that got me home by 5:00 p.m. every day and paid me just enough to buy a yard to mow with a house on it, raise a bunch of kids and lose some money playing golf every now and again. As long as my family was doing well I was going to be content.

When my principal project at work had stalled and rumors spread that it could be canceled, I started to get antsy. It occurred to me that I might not be able to sit still in my contented little world forever. There was mention of some job openings in a different division for the same company up in Philadelphia. That sounded rather intriguing, so I interviewed for one of the positions and they said they wanted to hire me. Damn, I hate when that happens. Lisa and I were both born and bred in the moderately paced Midwest and had spent the last eight years in the slower paced South. I decided it was time to give our life a jolt and move to the East Coast.

It was not easy to convince Lisa that it would be good for us to leave the comfortable country lifestyle we had built over the past eight years and start all over in a place that would prove to be completely different. She was well connected in the mommy network, had made some good friends, and she would have been content to stay there until all the kids had grown up. But I was ready for a change. I convinced Lisa and myself that this move would be good for my career and our family. Lisa trusted me and ultimately wanted me to be happy. She was going to be happy anywhere as long as we were all together. SOLD. So off we went, in the name of "Chris needs a change," to the fast-paced, car-filled, high-priced, land of the Northeast.

We felt uncomfortable from the start. Finding a decent house in our price range was almost impossible and we eventually settled for a home in Delaware, which meant I had to commute up I-95 to Philly every day. I-95 is an accident waiting to happen and when it does you can forget about getting home in less than an hour.

One night when I was working late a woman (who was later reported to have been on drugs) made the mistake of trying to walk from one side of the interstate to the other and got hit by a tour bus. At the time I did not know what had happened but all I knew

27

was that my highway home was completely closed for hours while the authorities cleaned up the mess. I tried to find an alternate route and wound up in a part of town that truly made me scared for my life. This was one time when not stopping to ask for directions was a desirable male trait and definitely the right thing to do. Not only did I not stop for directions, I did not stop for stop signs or red lights as I tried frantically to retrace my tracks. It was definitely in my best interest to wait so I could take my old friend, I-95, home.

When I finally walked into my house, Lisa (who had gotten used to me getting caught in traffic) had apparently dared to watch the Philadelphia news that night and knew about the accident on the highway. This place made her nervous. She didn't come right out and say it but when Lisa started wearing her ruby red slippers and chanting, "There's no place like home, there's no place like home," I figured she wanted to get out of there. I understood that the idea of living in Kansas and being close to her family was looking more and more appealing to her.

Despite our mutual concerns, we eventually worked into a routine that felt reasonably comfortable to us. The yard I had to mow was not as big as the one in Alabama, but I adopted a good chunk of the land owned by the utility company so I could get in more mowing time. Lisa was working the school system real hard and Samantha, our oldest daughter, was having a great year in kindergarten. Lisa had also made a couple of good friends and was getting networked in with the area and the other moms. As long as she had all the kid stuff under control, I was able to concentrate on my work and the lawn.

One morning my daughter Emily was running a fever and had been for three consecutive days. All good moms know that three is the maximum number of days to wait before taking a child to the doctor for a fever. Lisa asked me if I would be able to take off work and run her to our pediatrician. "We have a pediatrician?" This is when I found out that kids have to get physicals before they can go to kindergarten and that my insurance plan requires that we identify our children's primary care doctor. Fat, dumb and happy seemed to be working quite well for me at that point.

Career-wise things in Philly were going along pretty smoothly. My job was building some momentum, as I had moved into a manager's position with a group of about a dozen people under my supervision. Of course, with the added responsibility came longer work hours. The longer hours coupled with the unpredictable commute made a noticeable difference in the amount of quality time I was able to spend at home. My boss told me that if I continued to work hard he would push to get me promoted. This would mean a big bump in salary but also would mean a big bump in the stress and time required.

I had been to this point in my career a couple of times

before but I could never bring myself to the level of commitment required to play the corporate games full-tilt. But with Lisa staying home with the kids, it was my job to make sure that we were financially sound and to provide our kids with the opportunities that we thought were important for them. So I decided to give this career stuff another shot.

Even with all the positive things that we had going, the congested East Coast still made us feel uncomfortable and some-times unsafe. Maybe it was from watching the Philly news, which was like watching a war movie. Maybe it was that we were hundreds of miles away from the rest of our families. For whatever reason, somehow we knew that we would not be here forever and that something would happen that would take us away from this experiment of mine.

Lisa had been noticing a lump in one of her breasts, which was common for her each time she stopped breast-feeding. Just as a precaution she had a mammogram and was basically told, "Don't worry, no problem." About five months later the lump had grown a bit and an open sore had developed on her breast where the lump was located. We were both totally ignorant about such things, especially me. It never crossed my mind that this could be cancer. That just could not happen to us, right? Again, to be on the safe side, Lisa scheduled an appointment with a surgeon to have a biopsy performed on the lump.

"Hey, do you want me to go with you? It would give me a good excuse to get out of that weekly meeting that I love so much."

"No, you don't need to miss any work for this," she said quickly.

"The only thing I will be missing is my afternoon nap and the embarrassment of drooling on myself."

"No, really, I'll be fine. It's like going to the dentist. He'll just numb me up and cut out a chunk and that will be that," she said with a slight twinge of uncertainty, which I should not have ignored.

Our next door neighbor was going to watch the kids for us so I said, "Okay, but be sure to call me and let me know how it goes. If you change your mind later and want me to go, just call me."

"Just go to work and stop worrying," she said finally.

I was actually a bit relieved not to be going because I didn't like sitting around doctor's offices. But then who does? So me, Mr. Fat, Dumb and Happy, went skipping off to my little job up in the big city, not worried, but thinking it would be a good thing when it's over so we could put it behind us. The doctor probably would prescribe an ointment to take care of her skin irritation and that would be it. No shit, that's what I was thinking. Fat, REALLY dumb, and happy.

Her appointment was in the afternoon. I was sitting at my desk after lunch and my stomach started to knot up. At first I thought that my peanut butter and raisin sandwich had gotten stuck somewhere. As the time of her appointment ticked closer, my apprehension grew, and I finally decided that I would knock off early and head home. As I headed down I-95, a dark cloudbank that was shaped like a giant farm animal started to roll in. It got so dark that I had to turn on my headlights and by the time I pulled into my driveway it had started to rain.

The house was dark and I found Lisa sitting on the futon in the den. She was slouched over, her hands were clenched tightly between her knees and her eyes were red and droopy. Right then I knew that I should have been with her and I will never forgive myself for being so damn dumb. She rolled her eyes up to meet mine as the rain started pinging off the sliding glass door behind her. Raindrops welled up in her eyes like a storm cloud and then the bottom dropped out. "I have cancer," was all she said. This farm animal-shaped storm cloud was a cow, the cancer cow, and it ate us up.

We just sat there. I wrapped my arm around her while she sobbed uncontrollably and her tears fell as hard as the rainstorm outside. As she shrunk in my arms some of the highlights of our life together flashed before me. I remembered when this bright, blue-eyed girl bopped into work with her

"Party Time" hat on right after she bought her new red sports car. She was ready to conquer the world. Then I remembered her disappointment when she discovered how unfairly women were treated in the workplace. I remembered when we used to train for triathlons together and how impressed I was with her ability to keep up with me on our bikes. Years later she would confess that she hated riding with me, and that the only reason she did it was because she thought it was a quality I admired. She could chug a beer as fast as anyone, which was a quality I admired. I could see her as she bodysurfed in the Gulf and snow skied in the Rockies. I saw the agony of each of her four labors followed by the joy after each child was placed in her arms. I saw her as she dedicated her body and her life over the past eight years to having babies and taking care of them. We had talked about getting to the point where the kids would all be out of diapers and in school. Then she could get her body back in shape and we could move on to a new phase in our life. Now I saw that our future plans were all in jeopardy. I had no idea what would come next.

Then as quick as the storm blew in it blew out, and Lisa wiped the tears off her face. The mom kicked back in, and she announced, "I have to get the kids."

"Here, let me go get them, you can stay here and relax."

"Relax, how can I relax? I just found out I have cancer!"

Kids don't stop being kids just because you are sick.

Nothing stops, the world keeps spinning no matter what happens. Moms don't stop being moms, and in Lisa's case it became her sole mission for the rest of her life.

What happened immediately after the diagnosis was what I would call one of those 'cluster f #@!#' things. Panic was the word for the day as we started calling family and friends in an attempt to figure out what in the hell we were supposed to do. The surgeon she had seen for the biopsy was so sure it was cancer that he was ready to schedule a mastectomy even before he received the lab results. We met with him the next morning, and I could tell by the look in his eyes and his anxious tone that what he had seen in her was something very bad. He would not have made a good poker player.

The view from inside the cow was like looking through both ends of a telescope. Little things that used to be right in front of my face, which I had always taken for granted were suddenly so far away that I could barely see them. Things like standing in the kitchen and laughing about our neighbor's juicy phone conversation we had picked up on our baby monitor, or planning next summer's vacation. Other things that I could never see before were now becoming very visible and painfully clear, such as hospitals and death. Since I had been old enough to remember, no one in my family had died, and I had never known anyone else who had died. I had been sheltered from death and illness my whole life, and now

I found myself sloshing around inside of one of death's many stomachs contemplating how and when to break this news to our children.

"We don't know enough about what's going to happen yet to tell the kids. I wouldn't even know what to say," I said honestly.

"I want them in this from the beginning, and as we know more they know more. The longer we put this off the harder its going to be," Lisa said in a way that let me know she was going to do it regardless of my objections.

We gathered the kids together after dinner for what was going to be the first of the many talks that we never dreamed we'd have with our children.

"I went to the doctor today to see why I have this lump in my breast, and he told me that I have a disease called cancer," Lisa stated as calmly as possible. "I need to go see the doctor again to find out what they are going to do to make me better, so Grandma and Grandpa will be coming to help take care of you guys."

"What is cancer? My teacher told us that her sister has cancer and is very sick," said Samantha as she wrinkled up her forehead and scrunched up her nose.

"Your body is made of a whole bunch of tiny things called cells. Sometimes cells turn bad and start eating up the good cells. The bad cells are the cancer. The doctors have to find a way to get rid of the cancer cells so that they don't eat too many of the good cells," I said trying not to confuse them any further.

"We don't know much about it yet, so don't be scared. I just wanted you to know that cancer can make people very sick," Lisa told them bluntly.

Shyly, Emily raised her hand politely asking for permission to speak, "What does cancer look like? Can we see it?"

Lisa pulled the front of her shirt down far enough to see the bandage on the top part of her breast. She pulled the bandage back revealing the open wound caused by the tumor. All four of the kid's eyes went wide and they made a painful "Ooh ick" kind of face.

"Can people die from cancer," asked Samantha obviously afraid to hear the answer.

"Yes, sometimes if it is a really bad cancer the doctors and medicines can't fix it and people die," she replied.

"Are you going to die," asked Emily in a whisper.

"Nope, right now I'm fine and going to keep taking care of you just like always. So please don't worry about it. Okay?"

They all nodded.

"Now, who wants a sundae?"

The cancer cow was too fat to jump over the moon but our fat, dumb and happy bowl of ice cream life was running off with the spoon.

A Three Ring Circus

When I walked into my boss's office that morning I really wasn't sure what I was going to say. All I knew was that I had to tell him. I had to tell him that my life had changed, and that it was going to somehow affect my work. But I didn't know how or for how long.

Bill, my boss, was one of the smartest people I knew. He was an egghead mathematician with a very good grasp on what was important in life. The two of us would eventually become very good friends, as through our numerous talks we discovered that we shared many of the same values and beliefs. I believe that one of the biggest reasons that he offered me a job was because I went to a college he had almost attended because of its reported lack of racial prejudices. He had figured me as someone who didn't care about the color of his skin and he was right.

On this day, what I had to say would put a whole new perspective on what we talked about. "Hey, boss man," he said as I entered his gourmet coffee-scented office. He always called me "boss man" or "chief." It was his way of letting me know that he didn't think that because he was my manager he was automatically my superior. Bill would often preface a statement that was intuitively smart with, "I'm not all that smart, but . . ." This was his way of pointing out what should be obvious to people, without sounding like a know-it-all.

"My wife has breast cancer," I said in a poorly rehearsed tone as I sat myself down in a spare chair.

He started rubbing the bristled top of his head, which he did when trying to process information in his mathematical mind. "Cancer, man that is horrible. How old is your wife?"

"She's only thirty four."

"That's how old my wife is. Is it bad or do you know yet," he asked as he sat down stirring his coffee.

"Bad enough that the doctor who did the biopsy wanted to schedule a mastectomy before he even got the lab results back." Bill sipped his coffee and said, "Seems a bit hasty, but I don't know much about this stuff."

"Yeah, it scared the shit out of us. We wanted to talk to him more about it first. We have no idea what in the hell we are doing," I said as I paced back and forth in his small office.

Bill rubbed his head again and then stopped, meaning that he had completed his calculations. "I'm not a very smart man, but I do know that your family comes before anything. Whatever you need to do, just do it and I will make sure that no one around here gives you a hard time about it."

The significance of what he had said was enormous. He basically gave me a blank, paid leave of absence check, so that whenever I had to be gone for doctor appointments or family functions he was going to rubber stamp it. That was a tremendous load off my mind and would play a very big part in my ability to help my wife and family in the chemotherapy-ridden road ahead. We chatted uneasily for a few more minutes and then I immediately made a withdrawal from my new account. "I have to leave to meet my wife for our appointment with the surgeon. I will probably be gone the rest of the day."

"Do whatever you need to do, this place isn't going nowhere," Bill said, making good on his offer.

What had happened in Bill's office that morning was the beginning of a long line of nice things that people would do for my family and me. One of the silver linings in this cow-shaped storm cloud had been my discovery that in general, people are good. Most folks are genuinely eager to help someone in need. There are those who know what to do without having to be asked and there are those who are willing but have no clue what would be helpful. I eventually learned to seek out both of these types of people and ask for things that I never would have dreamt of asking for in my previous life. A certain power came with being a young man with

39

a job, four small children and a wife with cancer. It was a power that made people willing to do almost anything, sometimes without even being asked. Right or wrong, the only way I was going to manage this three-ring circus of family, job and cancer was to use and at times abuse this power.

Our meeting with the surgeon the day following the biopsy scared us out of our naive little wits. The talk of a rush mastectomy sent us scurrying home with our protective bubble ripped to shreds. We were in a panic mode and needed someone who could help us decide what we should do. We got on the phone and started calling our family and friends.

My brother, who lived down the coast in North Carolina, gave us the name and number of a radiologist friend who said he would be more than happy to talk with us. Lisa called him and they talked for well over an hour. She found out some of the basics about her disease that no one had taken the time to tell her. Things like what metastatic disease and aggressive stage IV tumors meant. Things that she didn't like but needed to hear. Here again was a person with his own wife and kids who took the time to talk with a complete stranger about some very uncomfortable and hard things. Three weeks after this phone conversation his wife would be eaten by the same cow, as she was diagnosed with the same type of cancer as Lisa's. These two women became almost instanta-neously bonded into a very close friendship. Reality seemed to be coming in piles of giant cow chips.

Exhausted from the emotional strain of relaying the bad news over and over again, we finally sat down at the kitchen table, nowhere nearer to a plan than when we started. If anything, we were more confused because of the different suggestions and opinions offered over the course of the day. At about 10:00 p.m. the phone rang. It was George, our pastor from Kansas, who was a long time friend of Lisa's family. He called to offer any kind of assistance or comfort that he could. George had recently been through surgery and treatments for prostate cancer, and spoke with the voice of someone who had been there and done that. His calming advice was simple, and temporarily made everything clear. "Hey guys, Lisa's mom and dad told me the horrible news. How are you holding up?"

"Not so good. We are really scared and have no idea what we should do. The doctor I saw thinks I need surgery right away, but I'm not sure," repeated Lisa.

"The one thing I learned through my experience is not to panic. People have a tendency in these types of situations to panic and make decisions that often end up being mistakes," George said in his convincing preacher's voice.

"It's too late George, we are already panicking and this surgeon is waiting for our decision. We don't know what to tell him," I said with obvious frustration.

"The thing you guys need to realize is that you live in a part of the country that has some of the best medical centers in the world. You owe it to yourselves to call one of these places and get a second opinion," he said thoughtfully.

At this point my kids would have said "Duh Dad," and if George was like my boss Bill, he would have prefaced his comments with "I'm not a very smart man but,......."

Lisa's uncle was tied into the medical industry and knew of a cancer center in Philadelphia that was supposed to be one of the best, so after a fitful night of sleep we called to make an appointment. There were some good vibes coming from this place even from the very first phone call. We could tell that they really knew what they were doing, and that this was where we needed to be. Then the reality that we weren't unique or even first in line at that institution began to intrude. The first available appointment to see a doctor was ten days away. When they gave me the date I was truly in a state of disbelief. How could they possibly expect someone with an aggressive stage IV tumor to sit patiently for ten days while the cancer continued to run unchecked? This was the drawback of going to one of the best cancer centers in the country, as it was obviously a very popular place. It was also the beginning of the end of my ignorance about a lot of things. In this case, it was discovering that the cancer cow had run amuck and was having its way with all kinds of people, even people like us who thought we were inedible.

Up to that point those were the longest days of our young lives, surpassing those long days of waiting for babies to make their entrance. There would be many more "longest days of our lives" yet to come, as playing a waiting game is the nature of this beast. We watched the clock tick. One night in the darkness of our bedroom she whispered, "I can feel it move."

"Feel what move," I whispered back.

"The cancer," she said, "I can feel it moving inside of me."

"What does it feel like?"

She put her hands on her chest, "It's hot like fire and it burns me inside as it moves." She grabbed my hand and placed it on her chest. "Can you feel how hot it is?" Then she started to cry.

"It's going to be okay," I said for the hundredth time that day.

"Well, what if it's not okay? How much farther is it spreading while we wait for that stupid appointment? At least the surgery would be doing something rather than waiting. I want this breast off of me."

The day of our appointment finally came. Lisa's parents had flown in from Kansas to help out with the kids and to be there for their daughter. They were relentlessly unselfish, and would end up spending most of the next 12 months living at our house. I went to work at about 5:30 a.m. to get in a couple of hours at the office before our trip into Philly. Then I drove back home, picked up Lisa and headed right back up I-95. The drive from our house was about 50 miles one way, but part of it was through an old section of Philadelphia and tended to be kind of slow. It took around 70 minutes to reach the cancer center. The building was much smaller than I had expected and was tucked away on the backside of a beautifully wooded city park. As we drove past the park for this first time I thought it would be a nice place to take a walk or run. My thoughts proved to be insightful, as in the months ahead, this park would become my safe haven. It was the place I would go for hours at a time, walking with my head close to the ground attempting to escape the reality of sickness that was all too common inside the walls of this place where I was a minority. A minority simply because I was not sick or dying. I felt no bond with the other non-dying spouses, as I always felt that somehow I wasn't supposed to be there. "No thanks, this is just a bad dream which will be over very soon and we will have our fat, dumb and happy life back again." In my case misery did not want company. It just wanted to be left alone.

This first appointment lasted most of the day. We were assigned to a team of "ist" people, and we met each one separately. We felt better about our decision to delay the surgery and wait for this appointment when the doctor told us that having surgery would have been a huge mistake. "Surgery will be one of the last steps in your treatment," assured Lisa's doctor. "We need the tumor intact so they we can easily gauge whether the chemotherapy is effective." In other words, there is no point in doing surgery if she doesn't survive the cow poison treatments. They took pictures of Lisa inside and out, including a Polaroid of her infected breast. When it was all said and done we had to set up another appointment to find out what kind of treatments she was going to need. Lisa tried to be brave but she was so scared and disillusioned that she started looking to me to make the rational decisions that a more secure Lisa would have made quickly for herself. When the doctor asked Lisa to sign a consent form to be a part of a study for the drugs she was going to get she said, "I don't want to be a guinea pig for a study. I want you to give me something that you know works." They tried to explain that because no one knows what works, everyone is part of a study. She finally gave up and looked to me to make the decision. My role as decision-maker would increase as time went on.

From that point forward, our lives were to be dictated by the cow and the cow fighters. Everyone else had to understand that they were second, including our kids and my coworkers. As sensible as that approach sounds, however, the truth is that all the understanding in the world won't freeze time. There came a point when the month-end report had to be completed, the yard needed to be mowed, and the insurance forms had to be mailed in. The grandparents would eventually need a break and have to go home, the children always needed someone to read to them and someone to take them to the park. Try as I might, I just could not get the world to stop or even slow down so that we could get our life straightened out.

Initially, Lisa's treatments had no impact on her tumor. In fact, the tumor continued to grow and they told us that at this rate she might last a couple of months. Lisa started to cry and said while shaking uncontrollably, "What about Thanksgiving and Christmas?" All she could think about was how her dying would ruin the holidays for her babies. I had no soothing words that made any sense, but that didn't stop my nervous, detached mouth from speaking. "Don't worry, everything will be fine."

"How can you say everything will be fine when I'm going to die?" I was reminded of one of the Astronaut Candidates 10 Commandments that I had pinned on my wall at work, which reads "Nothing is sometimes a good thing to do and always a clever thing to say."

When we got home from this doomsday appointment we told Lisa's parents the news. You could almost hear the air rush out of her mom, who seemed to shrink right before my eyes. She looked at her daughter through tear-filled eyes and said, "It should have been me, it should have been me."

It sounds like a line from a movie, but I assure you that

this is a real feeling that mothers have for their children. I started to think about this concept more logically and what I came up with was that I would have been a much better candidate to take this on. First of all, it should never be the mother. Mothers seem to have that extra dimension that I can't even describe, but I know it is there because I can feel it with my mom and I can sense it with our kids and Lisa. Lisa was by far the better parent between the two of us. She always had the right priorities when it came to our kids. My priorities were suspect and needed some work. She innately knew how to take better care of the kids than I did and had been the primary caregiver for their entire lives.

I had my reasons for feeling like I would be the more appropriate cancer patient. For one, I have a very high tolerance for pain and discomfort....almost disturbingly high. I have always treated pain as an emotion that can be shut off by the brain. A friend of mine and I would each eat three ice cream sandwiches on a hot summer afternoon and then run around the golf course until one of us puked. Or like when I spent half a day laying on my back in a mud filled trench as I held the jack hammer bit up with my feet with the handle resting on my stomach in an attempt to pound through a cement wall. This might be more an indication that not all my wires were connected, which might be a plus for the role of cancer patient. Every time I saw how much pain Lisa was in, I wished I could take it for her. My physical conditioning also gave me an advantage over Lisa. Not that Lisa was unfit (because the contrary was true) but exercising was an obsession of mine and might allow my body to better handle the brutal chemotherapy treatments. Maybe my most important credential was the fact that I had life insurance and she didn't. If I died she could afford to stay home and take care of the kids full-time. I, on the other hand, would have to continue to work and find others to take care of the kids when I couldn't be there.

Unfortunately life is not that way. We don't get to make those choices. One day George visited Lisa in the hospital and she asked, "George, how could God allow this to happen? Am I being punished?"

George said assuredly, "God has greater things in mind for you Lisa."

She said, "That's a bunch of crap. All I want to do is be a mother and raise my children. What could be more important than raising your children?"

The thought of dying in Philadelphia really bothered Lisa. "I can't die here. This place is cold and so far away from everyone. I want to be in Kansas, that's my home." The reality of the situation was that my job was not in Kansas, and I could not just quit because I needed the insurance provided through my employer to pay the bills.

"Well, I guess I could see if there are any job openings in

the Kansas division that I could apply for," I said realizing that those kinds of deals usually took more time to work out than what Lisa had. I was feeling stuck, and a little helpless, when some forces were put into motion on my behalf at work. A couple of days after Lisa made her plea, Bill called me into his office and told me that his boss had received a call from one of the Vice Presidents from the division in Kansas.

"Hey Boss Man," Bill said with a grin, "your father-in-law must have some high up connections because they said that any-time you need to relocate to Kansas they would find you a job and move you." Apparently, Lisa's dad made use of his forty years with the company and had called one of his many buddies. The next thing I knew I had a standing invitation for a job whenever I wanted it. It reaffirmed my faith in people and made me realize that regardless of a company's size, it is still made up of individuals who are good and want to do nice things for others. It also reminded me that who you know can sometimes make the differ-ence.

Later that week I was on the phone to the Human Re-source Department in Kansas to find out exactly how this potential move was going to work. I started getting my mind set on leaving Philadelphia, whose rat-race atmosphere I occasionally blamed for Lisa's illness. Philadelphia was a big place that undoubtedly had been blamed for a lot of other stuff, and since no one could tell us how a perfectly healthy body had contracted this disease it was as good a target as any for the blame I sometimes needed to place. On the flip side, I realized that Lisa might have had cancer before we left Alabama, and that we were fortunate to have moved to an area that was loaded with some really good "ists". Bill was sure that I was going to leave and started making plans to replace me.

At that point, the thought of going back to Kansas and to family was more than comforting, it was potentially life saving. Possibly for Lisa, but definitely for the kids and me. There was no way we were going to get through the whole ordeal without some serious family support. Then, just as we were finalizing our plans to move, things changed. As a last ditch effort, the doctors had tried a different kind of cow poison to see if it would do any good, and a small miracle occurred. We started to see with our naked eyes that the tumor was shrinking and the sores on her skin were starting to heal. I ran back to work. "Bill, don't give my job away. I still need it for awhile."

Now that they had the cow on the run, it didn't make sense to leave the care of these doctors and this reputable facility. Lisa had some hope for the first time, and wanted to wait until after all the treatments and surgeries were done before heading back to Kansas. It was difficult for me switching gears, but as the ringmaster I could only repeat, "The show must go on."

Over the next ten months I made so many round trips

(from work, to home, to the cancer center, back home and then back to work) that it makes my head spin to think about it now. I did not know how many hours of work I missed, but Bill never made an issue out of it. There were others, however, who weren't so understanding. They grew tired of my excuse for having to leave for this reason or that, not being able to support a meeting or take the time to look into a problem. The pressures at work were starting to build, and as I was staring down the barrel of a long, drawn-out treatment schedule I had serious doubts about my ability to keep the circus tent from falling on my already throbbing head.

There was one woman who worked for me who was more concerned for my family's well being than she was about the trivial things at work. She was a grandmotherly type who reminded me of Edith from "All in the Family." She cornered me one day at work and in a secretive whisper asked me, "Would you like some Holy Water?"

"Well, I don't know, why do you ask," I said curiously.

"I'm going to the Wailing Wall over Christmas and I can get you some authentic Holy Water for your wife," she said so no one else could hear her secret.

At this point I was looking for miracles so I said, "Sure, that would be great."

With all the holiday stuff going on at our house I had forgotten about the Holy Water deal I had made until I saw her approaching me on the first day back to work after New Year's. She walked up to my desk carrying a small, brown paper bag and handed it to me like she was making a drug deal. She didn't say a word and as she was leaving I said, "Thanks." Paul, the snoop sister I shared an office with, couldn't help but notice this bizarre little exchange and asked, "What's in the sack?"

"It's Holy Water. She brought it for my wife."

In his strong northeastern accent Paul asked, "Can I have a shot of dat der Holy Water in my coffee? I can use all the help I can get."

Inside the bag was a box containing six small glass bottles of water with little black, screw-on lids. When I got home I gave the bag to Lisa and told her what was in it. She opened the box, looked at the water and said, "What am I supposed to do with this?"

"I don't know. It didn't come with any instructions."

Shaking her head she tossed the box on top of the dresser and let it sit there for a couple of weeks. Then one morning as I was getting ready for work she opened the box and placed the six small bottles out in a row on top of the dresser. Then one by one she chugged the Holy Water like she was doing a round of shots at a bar. When they were all gone she wiped her mouth with her sleeve. She looked over at me as I stood there with my mouth hanging open and she said, "They say when you go overseas not to drink the water, but how bad can it hurt me at this point?" It had dawned on me that the reason she had waited to drink the water was to allow her chemo-depleted white blood cells time to build back up. She still wasn't taking any chances.

After she left the room I walked over to the empty bottles and shook the last drops out of each one into my mouth and dabbed a couple of drops behind each ear and one on the tip of my nose just for the hell of it.

It was a long, dreary winter of trips into Philadelphia for treatments that took eight hours each. I went to every one and stayed for the whole day. While we were gone the kids stayed home in the care of their grandparents, who were two of the strongest and most levelheaded people I had ever known. Their presence in our house was a great comfort. But this situation put a huge strain on them as they were forced to become the main caregivers for their daughter's kids instead of the spoiling grandparents that they wanted to be. When we would get home late in the evening, Lisa would be so tired and sick that she would go straight to bed. The kids would run and cling to my legs and neck and her parents would breathe a big sigh of relief that I was home so they could sit down and rest. Taking care of four kids all under the age of six is an all-consuming job that is both mentally and physically exhausting.

Each time I walked in the door after spending the day with Lisa at the hospital, I couldn't help but wonder if her parents resented the fact that I was spending these days with their daughter and they were not. Wasn't she their own flesh and blood? If Lisa had asked me to stay home with the kids and let her parents take her to her treatments, I would have obeyed. But I would not have liked it any more than her parents did. No matter how I looked at it, this was a losing situation for us all.

As the months dragged on, I began to feel like a stranger in my own house. There were almost always visitors staying to help out. When Lisa's parents weren't there, my parents, or Lisa's sister, or a friend would show up. It's not that I didn't appreciate the help. I just resented the fact that I needed it.

If I may be allowed to whine about one thing, it would be the invasion of my early morning privacy. Being a morning person, I really enjoyed waking up early and spending some very quiet time by myself to drink a cup of coffee, read the sports page, use my favorite downstairs bathroom and eat a bowl of cereal. Lisa's dad and my dad are both early risers as well, so this small niche of time I had once called my own had all but disappeared along with my private bathroom and unread sports page. Still, I really had no right to complain. My small inconveniences were nothing compared to theirs, as they weren't even in their own home. They never gave their dislocation a thought because they would unselfishly endure anything to help our family. I learned not to complain about anything because my worst "hardship" was nothing more than a hangnail compared to what Lisa had to put up with. The "I" and "me" in my list of frequently used vocabulary words had started to drop to the bottom of the page.

Only about one week out of four did Lisa feel okay and not have any scheduled doctor appointments. Occasionally this would be a week when there were no visitors because we could handle things ourselves. For those brief intervals, I felt back in control of my house and my family. Every morning was like Christmas. Of course the neighbors knew when there weren't any helpers around, and they would pick this time to strike with the delivery of food. One woman in particular would bring us dinner with so much food she had to wheel it up the street to us in a very squeaky little red wagon. We could hear her coming all the way up the hill and so could the rest of the neighborhood. Everyone knew that the needy Donner family was getting a meal. She dropped the squeaky meal wagon off in our garage and told me that I could return it at my convenience. I wanted to tell her to stop bringing stuff but she was acting out of genuine kindness. And she was the only person who thought to bring me beer.

The first time I returned the wagon, I walked with an awkward slouch (because the handle was to short) and the wagon was squeaking so loudly that I imagined everyone peering out their windows to look at the poor guy with the sick wife. The next couple of trips I purposely made late at night, carrying the wagon

55

the whole way.

It was also during those good weeks that Lisa and I would get reacquainted with our children. They re-energized us with their laughter, playfulness and unconditional love that had survived undamaged by the harsh experiences and realizations that come with cancer. How long would it be before their protective bubbles burst? I wanted to believe that their innocence was still intact, but realistically some of it had to have been altered or lost completely to the cow.

The logistics of Lisa's treatment schedule became even more complicated when, because of her good progress, she became eligible for a stem cell transplant. For this procedure Lisa was put in the hospital for weeks, loaded up with toxic chemicals basically designed to kill everything good and bad in her body, and then infused with her own blood cells through her spine. The hope was that the transplanted stem cells would start to grow and replenish her body.

Every day for the five solid weeks of her stay in the hospital, I went and visited her. Three of those weeks she was so doped up on morphine that she either slept through my entire visit or couldn't remember that I had been there. To Lisa, those weeks never happened, which was a good thing. It was during those few weeks that I started to see things, kind of like when the Grinch heard all the Who's down in Whoville singing on Christmas morning. Actually, it wasn't seeing as much as developing a feeling for what's really important, or understanding things at some higher level. The idea of "getting it," like the Grinch finally got "it" about Christmas. He finally understood (or felt) that Christmas wasn't about the presents, but was a celebration of Life. As the story goes, "His heart grew three sizes that day." As I sat in that hospital room looking at this shadow of a body, I could feel my heart grow as I was starting to get "it". We are forced to live inside the body we were given but the body is not who we are. Lisa was still there, undiminished, even though her body was giving out on her. Those who focus on the scarf-wrapped head instead of the person's eyes just can't be getting "it." Unfortunately this realization often comes only as the result of some tragic event, and is why people forced to face death (either personally or through someone close to them) are often the ones who are given this gift.

Time, I realized, was a very precious commodity. Spending an hour with my children was more important than making sure that my grass was a certain height. The time I spent visiting Lisa, even though she didn't acknowledge my presence, was more important than making sure someone at work was following the right procedure. It was as if I had gone from watching a 6-inch black and white T.V. to sitting in the front row of a wide-screened movie theater with color and surround sound. Once I got a glimpse of the big screen it was impossible to see images on the small one.

This awareness for me was both enlightening and dangerous. Dangerous because everything that wasn't in focus at this new higher level seemed so trivial, including my job. It became increasingly difficult for me to perform these now irrelevant tasks when I could be at home spending time with my family. My tolerance for people who in my opinion didn't get "it" was almost zero. I walked around with a chip on my shoulder, daring the non-IT people to knock it off. I think people could sense this, and in general they were a little bit afraid of me and left me alone.

For the five weeks Lisa was in the hospital, I managed to spend a little bit of time in each of the three rings of my circus. My daily schedule included about three hours of driving time. When I finally got home, I played with the kids while Lisa's mom and dad made dinner. Then I would get the kids bathed and put to bed. After the kids went to bed, I updated Lisa's parents on her condition which changed very little from day to day and started sounding like a broken record. Then they would read for a bit and sometimes dare to watch the news before going to bed. Usually I was keyed up for quite awhile, and rather enjoyed the quiet time as I swept the kitchen floor and did a load of wash. Going to bed was beginning to lose its appeal and started to feel like a waste of valuable time.

Just to make things more interesting, the battery on Lisa's dad's pacemaker started to give out and he found himself in the emergency room of Lisa's hospital. He ended up having surgery to install a new pacemaker and was in a room two floors above his daughter. Because the hospital was in a scary part of town, I felt it was best that I accompany Lisa's mom when she went to visit her husband and daughter. We were constantly scrambling to get babysitters. The kids didn't know who was coming or going anymore.

This crazy schedule finally made dealing with the pressures at work impossible, and something was going to have to give. Again I called on my newly found power to transform from a quiet, mild mannered boy into the bold and forceful "Super Cow Man." I asked my boss if I could be relieved of my supervisor position and become more of an individual contributor, meaning that I wouldn't have to worry about anyone except myself. He agreed and I found a nice, quiet, out of the way desk where I could slowly decompose without bothering anybody. I more than put my career on hold, I put it in reverse and hoped that I could somehow stay employed. I was counting on the compassion of those I worked for. The show in my three ring circus that I called my career had very few interested spectators, and I was finding it difficult to maintain some sort of balance as the cow was eating up more and more time.

One afternoon I was sitting in someone's office and noticed a quote taped to the cover of a notebook. The quote dealt with maintaining the proper balance in your life, and compared life to a game where you had to juggle your family, health, friends, and job.

It suggested that your job was a rubber ball that, if dropped, would bounce back. The other things, however, were said to be made of glass and would be irrevocably damaged if they were dropped. I was banking on that being true, as I was letting my career slip in the hope that it would bounce back, and putting most of my effort into keeping my family from hitting the ground. What I would find out was that my job, like a rubber ball, would bounce a little lower each time it hit the ground. Without a positive force the ball only has so many bounces before it stops and just lies there on the floor.

Lisa and I did our best to keep the day to day activities around our house as normal as possible. Even with the numerous treatment trips and the constant shuffling of visitors, we managed it quite well. There were times, of course, when things were just too far out in left field to pretend that everything was fine. Like those five consecutive weeks that Lisa was in the hospital and couldn't have any children as visitors. Or the period when the treatments weren't working, and swarms of relatives and friends came visiting from the four corners of the country because they were afraid that they would not see her alive again. It's very morbid watching people pay their last respects when the recipient is still very much alive. There was some added pressure in constantly being in the mode of host, but everyone was willing to pitch in and do their share of work. Also, the various visitors were giving Lisa and the kids some much needed extra attention that I was unable to give them, as I had to take every available moment to keep my job afloat.

With summer came the end of the treatments, tests and surgeries, as Lisa was considered to be in "remission." She was now ready to move back home to Kansas. All I had to do was call that person in the human resource office of the Kansas division and say, "Remember me? I'm the guy in Philadelphia you talked to five months ago whose wife was about to die and wanted to relocate to Kansas. Then we needed to wait because she started to get better. Now she is not about to die, well not yet anyway, and we would still like to move even though the company has started to down-size and currently has a hiring freeze," and so on. Super Cow Man's powers were being severely tested. I found myself making Lisa's present condition sound worse than it really was in hopes of drumming up some sympathy. I was careful not to use the word "remission" as this term to the layperson often means "cured." I didn't feel right doing this, but everyone was counting on me to make this happen and I was desperate.

The original momentum and sense of urgency had long since diminished. I was stuck trying to find an actual job vacancy, and then to convince someone to hire me. It got very complicated, and I had to work it for months before I finally found someone who had some budget and a job for which I was almost qualified. Basically, I was at the mercy of this huge company and would take

61

whatever job they offered. My reaffirmed faith in people was slightly dented by the realization that it is easy for someone at the top of the corporate heap to wave their wand and say, "Sure we can give him a job," then walk away leaving those all-important details for others. My rubber ball of a career was being dropped again on a floor covered with jagged rocks which could send it bouncing just about anywhere.

Meanwhile, Bill was once again so sure of my leaving that he stopped giving me any work. I was slowly fading into obscurity. Lisa was so sure that we were leaving that she asked her dad to send real estate guides so that she could begin house hunting. She also had found a new oncologist and started scheduling radiation treatments at the cancer center in Kansas. The kids were excited because they were sure that they were going to be living in a new house right next door to their grandparents. Lisa's parents were anxiously awaiting our arrival so they could be close to their daughter without being 1300 miles from home. Unfortunately, in my own stressed-out mind, I wasn't sure of anything except that my family was counting on me to get them back to Kansas and I hadn't figured out how to do that yet. "Hey Dorothy, how about forking over those damn ruby red slippers?"

Hope Runs Wild

For some reason my dad seemed to enjoy finding me jobs that no one else wanted. They usually required a certain mindless physical stamina and a willingness to do whatever was needed no matter how dirty, sweaty or disgusting. Maybe he recognized a certain tenacious quality in me, or maybe he just figured I wasn't very bright. Don't ask me why, but I did kind of enjoy that sort of work because the jobs usually gave me a good physical workout while at the same time allowing my mind to wander. My mom once told me that when I was little she would leave me sitting in the car for hours, (probably with the motor running), while she shopped. When she returned I was always sitting right where she left me, possibly a bit lethargic from the fumes, but content and drooling.

The kinds of jobs my dad landed for me included such things as pulling weeds for the city park department. I would literally pull weeds in flower gardens eight hours a day. Then there was a job building slurries on farms. Slurries are huge metal tanks used to store cow and pig manure so the farmers could make their own fertilizer. One sweltering summer day I spent hours down in this cement pit, knee deep in a soupy mixture of pig excrement and rainwater, in an attempt to retrieve all the small rocks off the bottom. When I came home in the evening my mom understandably made me eat outside on the screened porch. Then came a great job in a steel mill where I was a "heater." This involved loading and unloading fifty-pound steel bars from a 1700-degree open-hearth furnace. Another summer I ran a ninety-pound jackhammer for a month straight. Then I worked for a Rotor Rooter man where the kind of dirt that I had my hands in taught me not to chew my finger nails. Whenever someone asked, "How's business," I learned to respond by saying, "It's shitty." That was my day job. In the early, early morning I was one of those guys hanging off the side of a garbage truck dumping rat infested trash from the town's restaurants. That work spoiled my appetite for dining out at those establishments.

Unfortunately I could go on, but my point is that I had a certain personality trait which lent itself to this sort of activity and made me capable of handling the daily chores that came with the cancer cow. The frustration with my job as cow-puncher, however, came in not being able to see the end of the task. It was like being asked to clean the manure out of the cow's stall only to have the cow replace the piles as quickly as you shovel them out. There are only two ways this job could end. I either had to quit or the cow had to leave, neither of which was likely to happen anytime soon. There was no way I was going to quit.

When I was sixteen, my dad (who knew the owner of the town's only country club) worked out some kind of trade, and suddenly I was confronted with an "offer" to work the country club's Sunday morning brunch. Our family had eaten there on occasion, which meant that I should have known better and refused. As I think back on this brunch now, I conjure up an image of the food fight scene at the college cafeteria in the movie "Animal House." However, based on the way my dad was leaning on me to take this thankless, low paying job, I figured he had cut some deal with the owner to get a discount on the club membership fees. I accepted the job, mainly because someone asked me if I wanted it. I was easy.

At first the people trickled in and we greeted each other with a friendly hello and a smile. But it wasn't long before there were more people then there were seats, and I literally had to run as I cleared tables, cleaned up syrup spills and kept the buffet stocked. It was high-speed confusion as everywhere I turned someone was asking for or spilling something. As soon as a group got up to leave there was another group waiting to sit down. My patience with people grew short and I started finding it difficult to smile at anyone.

Then the hordes trickled back out, and almost without noticing I was once again walking instead of running. Where there were once wall to wall people I could now see table tops and empty chairs. My God, there were windows, the sun was shining, and guys with plaid pants were driving by in golf carts. Once again I was personable and pleasant. Clearing the tables became almost fun, as I could do it at my own pace. As I cleaned one and moved on to the next I knew I would not have to touch it again. As I watched the last family of farmers, a group of 23, walk out the door I heard the sound of coins falling out of the tip jar signifying that the end was near. I let out a big birthday candle sigh of relief.

In many ways this was the way it felt as Lisa and I fled, at a dead run, from the crowded, screaming tables of Philadelphia to the spacious, empty chairs and tables of Kansas. We loaded up our plum colored mini-van with enough supplies for a couple of weeks, set our compass west and headed out. Our house had not sold yet and we did not have a house of our own to move into, but there comes a point when you have to say "Screw it, let's go." Lisa had wanted to have her radiation treatments in Kansas, which is why we had to get her there before we were ready to move. Lisa's parents were going to be the lucky recipients of our presence, and were no doubt bracing themselves for the assault of four young children, a very sick daughter, a stressed out son-in-law and an overweight dog. This was truly an indication of their love and support for their daughter and her family. But as we drove across the country singing "The wheels on the bus go round and round," over and over again, none of that seemed to matter. All that did matter was that Lisa was in remission and she was going home. For the first time since the initial attack from the cancer cow there was a sense of hope.

The drive itself was over 1300 miles, which we had planned on making in two days. The most amazing thing about the drive was this feeling I had (which I am sure Lisa felt as well) that with each passing mile the weight and weariness of the past year was slowly lifting. "Hey, have you noticed that no one is passing us or honking and flipping us the bird. I might even be the fastest car on the highway," I said as I passed another mini-van.

Lisa smiled, "Yeah, and there is land that doesn't have houses and buildings on it."

"Back home we like to call that the countryside ma'am," I kidded.

She was in a more reflective mood. "The farther we get from that place the better I feel. It was so claustrophobic and depressing. I can take a deep breath without choking on it," she said as she demonstrated her breathing technique.

"I think everyone feels better," I said as I honked and waved at some horses that were grazing in an open field.

It was like driving in a pipe that started out very narrow

and dark and as we drove got wider and brighter. Still, it seemed as though we would never get completely out of that pipe. It was hot, we had been driving for two straight days, Dusty (our dog) was really starting to smell, or maybe it was me. I really couldn't tell anymore.

There were countless delays for road construction, and at one point we sat stranded on the blistering asphalt for over 45 minutes. The delays caused us to hit Kansas City during rush hour, but by then I had fire in my eyes and I put those Philadelphia driving skills to use. Every car on the road was the enemy as I raced faster and faster in my attempt to break free one last time. The roads went from eight lanes down to six and finally to four, as the number of cars once again dwindled like the diners at the end of that Sunday brunch. Then it happened. As we reached the top of a small rise we shot out of the end of the pipe like a cannonball and the explosion in front of us was the Flint Hills of Kansas. Lisa started to cry. We were speechless, as there were no words to describe what we felt at that moment. I doubt that she thought that she would ever get another chance to see this wide-open piece of Kansas that she had taken for granted her whole life. The hills were covered with nothing except for grass and the speckling of livestock for as far as the eye could see. On this day, at this moment, heaven stretched out before us. It was a moment of weightlessness, when the heavy burden of cancer was lifted and sucked out the open van window like one of the many loose candy wrappers.

As we rolled into town Lisa was pointing out familiar landmarks to the kids and noticing new housing developments and "For Sale" signs. The number one order of business was going to be finding a house. We knew that we could live with Lisa's parents for as long as we needed, but it wasn't going to be easy. It had been such a long time since we had any kind of normal existence that we were aching to get into our own place as soon as possible. The thought of having the opportunity to be boring was exciting.

We were still a long way from boring. Our house in Delaware was nowhere near being sold. There had been a contract on it, but it fell through a few weeks before the scheduled closing. My new job was not scheduled to begin for a couple of weeks, which meant I had to drop off Lisa and the kids, then turn around and drive all the way back to Delaware. It was actually a nice break for me, and even though the drive back by myself was kind of a bitch, it was still relaxing. Two solid weeks without kids, and without doctor appointments. It was just my house, my yard and me. Yes, I could actually mow my grass without having to rush, and when I was done I sat down on my back steps and had a beer. A rare respite indeed.

After months of begging, pleading and groveling I had found someone in the Kansas division willing to take me on and give me a job. My last day at my job in Philadelphia went without notice. Although I was glad to be leaving, it still made me sad because of the kindness everyone had shown to us. There were many emotions wrapped up in this place and the last thing I wanted was any kind of awkward going-away party. My boss, Mr. Bill, took me out that night and we went to places in downtown Philly that the average white dude did not know about. At one of the bars my name kept getting pulled out of a Moosehead beer hat that eventually qualified me for a one in twelve chance to win a new Jeep. Unfortunately, the drawing for the car was going to happen after I was gone and I had to be present to win. Oh well. My last night in Philadelphia finally ended. "Good luck to you and your family," Bill said as he extended his hand. "If you ever need anything just call me." Neither of us knew it at the time, but I would be taking him up on that offer later.

It was 100 degrees when the movers were loading up the truck. Because my plan was to get in the van as soon as the house was emptied and cleaned, I offered to help them so as to speed up the process. Finally, at about eight p.m., after being sweat-soaked and dried many times over, I jumped into the plum colored mini-van and slipped out of town never to be heard from (there) again. I drove all night and the next day, arriving at Lisa's parent's house in time for supper. The next morning I got up with blurry-eyed, caffeine-powered optimism, and started my new job.

Lisa's dad took her to all of her radiation treatments,

which were scheduled to be every day for a month if her body could tolerate it. They had drawn large X's on her body so that the "ists" with the ray guns would know where to shoot. The first couple of weeks went well but then her skin started to get burnt and very sore. The radiation made her nauseous and her already weakened body was barely able to tolerate this new abuse. What else could they do to this poor, battered woman? After months of chemotherapy, a stem cell transplant, a mastectomy and now radiation, I had to wonder if they realized that she was still a person. This was the only part of her treatment in which I did not directly participate.

When Lisa was not being radiated she was busy getting Samantha and Emily enrolled in school (second grade and kindergarten, respectively). She also was scouring the city and all the surrounding communities for houses so that we would be ready whenever our house in Delaware sold. Every house or lot we looked at had to be judged, in part, based on how long it took to get to her parent's home. She was not as optimistic as I was, and she was still planning for the worst and wanted her parents to be easily accessible. As time wore on, the search radius from her parent's house got smaller and smaller until I noticed that she began looking exclusively at houses in her parent's development. Their development was large, relatively new and out of our price range. But I could tell this was the place she was going to feel comfortable, so I started developing a creative financial plan, which counted heavily on winning the lottery.

If there was a record for enduring the most high stress situations simultaneously, I believe I would have been in the running. I was moving halfway across the country, selling a house, buying a house that I couldn't afford, dealing with mounting medical bills, starting a new career, living with my in-laws, helping manage four kids and a dog, caring for my sick wife and lacking a yard to mow. It would be unethical for one man (me) to ask another man (my father-in-law) to mow his lawn for him. I should have been about to explode. Instead, I was so full of hope that Lisa was going to make it that I was ready to endure anything based on that possibility.

Over the prior year I had grown weary of not knowing what was going to happen, not being able to see the end. Was she going to die or live? I couldn't imagine how she was able to face each day. Maybe she knew or had a sense, and had figured out a way to deal with her reality. I don't know. What I do know is that she was infinitely stronger than anyone I had ever known. For selfish reasons I wanted to know the outcome, so that I could move forward with my life. I must admit (and I will probably go straight to hell for this) that there were times when Lisa's condition was getting worse and I secretly wished she would just go ahead and die. It wasn't that I stopped caring, or that my love for her had diminished. The contrary was true, as my admiration for her grew each day as she continued to tolerate these unbearable conditions. But I had read too much and heard too many cancer horror stories. Deep down, in spite of my hopefulness, I had to know what the final outcome would be.

Before Lisa went into "remission," I found it frustrating when her test results would come back with little or no change from the previous test. Lisa would be grateful because she figured she had just bought herself more time to be with her kids. A part of me was actually disappointed because it meant more time in never-never land. There was always a big discussion involving the quality of life of the patient, which boiled down to whether the hell of more treatments with little hope for survival was worth it. Was the small chance of improvement really worth Lisa's feeling so physically ill that she could not enjoy her family, or would it be better to admit the inevitable, stop taking any toxic drugs, spend some quality time with her family and let nature take its course? What about the quality of our kids' lives, Lisa's parents' lives, and my life? Should we be factored into this quality of life equation? Our answer basically was "no." We felt that the quality of our lives would improve only if Lisa were to survive. At the time, continued treatments was the only option that offered any chance, as remote as it was. I had often wondered if Lisa's parents had ever wished for their daughter's suffering to end, but I was too ashamed to ask them.

The strain of our cohabitation with her parents was beginning to show on their faces and in their eyes, and I knew that something was going to have to change soon. I sensed we were about to hit the bottom of what I had thought to be a bottomless pit of never-tiring support. Then miraculously, our house sold, although because of our desperate situation we settled for less than we otherwise would have. After paying our real estate agent, we barely broke even. We didn't care because I was sure to win the lottery any day now, and we could finally start house hunting instead of window-shopping.

While waiting for the closing on the sale of the Delaware house, Lisa found the home of her limited dreams. "I found it," she said unable to hide her excitement.

"Found what," I asked playing the part of the dumb straight man.

"Our new house. It's perfect. It backs up to the park and the kids can walk or ride their bikes on a sidewalk to Mom and Dad's house. It's only a few blocks away. There is also a big garage and a basement," she added as if those two features would seal the deal.

"How big is the yard?" I asked playing along.

"It backs up to the park. You can mow that too if you want. Do you want to go see it?" Lisa asked as if I had a choice.

"You mean you haven't already bought it? Sure. When?"

"In an hour. I called the agent and set it up," she said with a big cheesy grin.

Looking at the home was only a formality, because I could tell how badly she really wanted that house. The trick was to come up with the cash to buy it. "Can we afford this house?" she asked, knowing that we couldn't.

"No, but if we use our retirement funds we could probably make it work," I said not knowing for a fact if it would.

Lisa gave me a look that told me she couldn't care less about retirement, as she figured that she would never get a chance to enjoy it. We made an offer on the spot and bought the house just before Thanksgiving. She was so excited that even though the house was filled with unpacked boxes, she insisted on having Thanksgiving dinner in our new nest. It was truly a joyous occasion for which we were genuinely thankful. Lisa broke a family tradition and said the grace instead of her father. With a trembling voice she prayed, "Thank you God for my truly wonderful family and blessing me with four beautiful and healthy children. And God bless Chris for buying me this house. Amen. Now let's eat."

The rest of her family seemed relieved to have us in town, as though this was where Lisa and the kids were supposed to be. As for me, I was content to stay right where we were because I knew it made everyone feel comfortable and safe, even though I personally felt slightly out of place.

Christmas was pretty much the same happy story, as we were able to spend it with her parents and brothers and sister who had all come to town for the holidays. Lisa had gone to great lengths to make sure that this was a perfect Christmas for the kids. Her persistent realism, which at times I resented, kept her from thinking that she would be around for many more holidays. She treated this one as if it would be her last. Every time she started to relax and really enjoy herself it would trigger a defense mechanism that reminded her of the odds against survival. The laughter would turn into an apprehensive smile and she would get back to the task of preparing for her departure. It was sad to watch, as I selfishly wanted to pretend that everything was fine, at least for a little while. I was trying to slip back into that fat, dumb and happy lifestyle that I desperately missed. As quickly as possible I was putting the past year behind me; our lives had been on hold long enough. I was marking off each day trying to get to that magical five-year remission mark that the 'ist' people say means there is a good chance of long-term survival. In my mind, each day that went by without relapse was equal to a dog's day. Hope is a double-edged sword that can be very dangerous when wielded by someone like myself, who refused to recognize the sharpness of both edges.

My job was turning out to be pretty decent, and under the circumstances was a darn good fit for me. They put me on a very unique project that no one knew exactly how to do. There were no right ways or wrong ways established, so it was all kind of loosey-goosey, which was perfect for the frame of mind I was in. Everyone in my new group had heard my story before I got there, which automatically put me out of their comfort zone (with the exception of my soon-to-be good friend Bruce). This was fine with me, as I no longer had the capacity to carry on idle chitchat with people that I really didn't know. It felt like such a waste of time.

No one was reporting to me, so the only person I had to worry about was myself. Bruce, who sat next to me, was an easygoing, funny guy. He was in charge of looking after his grandmother who was dying of brain cancer in a nursing home, which gave him a good understanding of the cow and made him very easy for me to talk to. Some days we would talk more than work. I'm sure that our boss was not happy with our relative lack of productivity, but she pretty much left me alone. Maybe she was afraid that I would crack and come in one day with a machine gun. Going to work started to be fun, and for the first time in a very long time I actually looked forward to each day.

The kids were cruising, almost as if nothing had ever happened. Their mom's hair had grown in, she didn't have to wear those masks anymore, and as far as they could tell she was no longer seeing any doctors. They had their mom back. Life was good.

Lisa was fairly upbeat and slowly had been getting some of her strength back. They told us that the drugs had in effect aged her body at least twenty years and she would never feel like she did before. She was a 35 year-old mother, with four kids, stuck in the body of a 60 year old. She was determined to get back in shape, and when she heard an advertisement for the Race for the Cure she immediately started training to run it.

The Race for the Cure is a walk/run fund-raiser for breast cancer and is held in cities all over the United States. Of course I had never heard of this event before, but during that fat, dumb and happy part of my life I was unaware of many things. One of the missions of the Race for the Cure is to promote breast cancer awareness, which I had learned the hard way. The whole family rallied behind Lisa as she tried to get in good enough shape to complete the 5K walk/run. She had a hard time running because she had almost no feeling in her feet as a result of all the nerve damage caused by the chemotherapy. Not being able to tell exactly where her toes were, she would constantly catch them on the ground and trip, a small inconvenience in exchange for her life. To the casual observer she just looked clumsy, but she really didn't care what anyone else thought. Her parents, the kids and myself all started training for the big run. It was the first positive thing we had done together in a long time.

The race started at 8:00 a.m. on a crisp, autumn day, and

everyone got up early with Christmas morning-like enthusiasm. We arrived early to get registered and pick up our race numbers, and were surprised at the large crowd and the party atmosphere. They had loud, up-beat music and a stage with a high-energy aerobics instructor leading a group of people in a pre-race warm up routine. The kids found a rainbow-striped tent that had tables of donuts, fruit and hot chocolate, making the event an instant success.

There were a couple of aspects of this race that really stood out. At the table where we picked up our race number (which was to be pinned on the front of our shirts) there were some large, thick sheets of pink paper. These pink sheets had written on them either the words, "In Support Of," or, "In Loving Memory Of," and were to be pinned to your back. Underneath those words was a bunch of blank pink space where you could write the name or names of the people you wanted to recognize. My kids thought this was very cool as they proudly wore their, "In Support Of MOM!!!" signs as if it were some kind of medal. These four little kids with their "MOM" signs covering their entire backs drew a lot of attention from the other participants, as there can be nothing more inspiring than the natural bravery of children.

My kids were downright bubbly as they walked around with donuts and drinks. I walked up to Samantha who was busy chatting with a stranger. "My mom is running in this race. She had breast cancer and can't feel her feet. That's her standing over their talking to my grandma," she said with her mouth full and pointing with her donut-filled hand. Watching and listening to her made it possible for me to start breathing easily again.

The easygoing camaraderie amongst strangers was the other interesting phenomenon I had noticed. There was a bond between all of us, like a single thread of understanding running through each of our hearts. It wasn't necessary for people to spend time talking about their cancer, their mom's cancer, or their wife's cancer. The fact that we were there indicated a certain level of knowing that did not need to be hashed out. What we all wanted was to embrace each other with hugs of understanding, smiles of hope, and words of encouragement. It was almost as if the fundraising for the fight against cancer was secondary, as I imagined this incandescent glow of hope that an aerial picture of this spectacle would certainly capture. Sometimes I felt invisible as I drifted in this sea of people, whose lives had been unexpectedly and permanently altered. I felt invisible because I couldn't fully accept that I was supposed to be there. This was the same feeling I had walking around the cancer center in Philadelphia. A huge part of me still denied that this had happened to us, to me.

The race was split into three separate events. The men ran first, then the women, and the fun run for kids was last. As I lined up for the start of the men's event, the pace of my heart started to gain momentum. There was a nervous sound of tennis shoe-covered hooves as the herd of runners jumped and jogged impatiently in place, waiting for the sound of the horn triggering the start of the stampede. By the time the horn finally blasted, my insides had already run the race at least once and were ready to go again. However, because I was not in the very front row I had to wait for the equivalent of that bizarre traffic light thing where all the cars can see that the light is green yet they all can't seem to start moving at the same time. I was still moving at a crawl when I went past my cheering kids, Lisa and her mom. The pack finally broke up and I was able to start running at what felt like a world record-setting pace. There was so much adrenaline pumping through my veins that I thought I could run like that forever, or at least for the first mile, whichever came first. The one-mile mark came first, and I found myself bent over, holding my gut, gasping for air. I pretended to be tying my shoe as eighty-year old Grandpas and pregnant-looking middle aged macho men with sleeveless shirts passed me. The shame overcame the pain and I managed to catch my breath enough to continue. Actually, I began thinking about all that Lisa had endured and overcome just so that she could be here, and what a wimp I was being in comparison. This is what inspiration is about, so I sucked it up and headed on down the road in Lisa's honor, bent on catching those old and pregnant guys.

Shortly after the conclusion of the men's race, the women starting lining up for their run/walk. This is when all the hootin' and hollerin' took place because standing in this group were women like Lisa who were survivors with supporters in the crowd. With my youngest daughter Gaven on my shoulders and the other kids at my side, we cheered as their mother jogged by waving and grinning like a high school prom queen.

As it neared the time when we thought she might be getting close to finishing, the kids and I found a seat on the curb so that we could cheer her on as she completed the last hundred yards to the finish line. We waited and waited. In my fat, dumb and happy mind I had underestimated, or failed to believe, the damage that had been done to her body. I apparently was still refusing to accept the reality of it all.

Because of the sharp curve in the road we couldn't see people coming until they were right on us, so when she came shuffling around the corner the kids almost missed her. One of them spotted her and shouted, and before I knew what had happened all the kids had run out into the street, oblivious to the other runners that they cut off as they grabbed onto their mom's arms and legs, screaming the whole time. Lisa could do nothing except stop or risk falling on top of them. The five of them stood tangled for a moment until Lisa grabbed them by their hands and started jogging with the four of them in tow. The other people watching started cheering. They understood the magnitude of what they were witnessing. The announcer at the finish line called out Lisa by name over the loud speaker, "Here comes Lisa Donner, a survivor, and it looks like she has a lot of help." There was a lump in my throat the size of a bowling ball as I choked back the tears. If I were a screenwriter and wanted to make a movie that ended with everyone feeling good and full of hope, I would end the movie just as this race ended. Mother and children, hand in hand, crossing the finish line with the crowds all cheering. Everyone in the theater would leave feeling fat, dumb and happy, just as I was beginning to feel once again.

Save the Children

Winters in Kansas seem tailor made for breeding colds and the flu. One day it might be 60 degrees and sunny and the next morning it's snowing with a minus 10 degree wind chill. These extremes must confuse the body's defenses and make it vulnerable to attacks from the armies of mindless microscopic critters. Then when you enter into the equation four snot-nosed children, who might as well be aircraft carriers for germs and bacteria, it is no wonder that there is always someone coughing, sneezing or vomiting. The cold and flu season appears to coincide with the holiday season, starting with someone throwing up on Halloween and then hitting every major holiday up through Easter.

Because Lisa's immune system had been permanently damaged by the chemical warfare, she was extra cautious and would often wear hospital masks whenever any of our kids were ill. Despite her efforts, it was inevitable that she would eventually catch a cold. Her cold started in the middle of January as just an annoying sniffle, which she could not shake and which was later joined by a small, nagging cough. "You really should go to the doctor and get something stronger for your cough," I suggested as Lisa sniffled by carrying the never-ending basket of laundry.

"It's just the same cold I get every winter. I'll be fine," she replied without breaking stride.

I followed her into the next room, "With your low blood counts you need to be careful or you will end up in the hospital with pneumonia."

"I'm not going to the doctor just so they can poke around and try to find something wrong. The last time I went in for a routine checkup I came home with cancer."

I couldn't blame her for her paranoia and didn't push it. Her regular monthly checkup with the oncologist was coming up in a few weeks so she opted to wait until then.

Her runny nose and cough persisted over the weeks, and if anything, got a bit worse. It seemed that whenever other people were around she tried to muffle her cough, hoping that nobody would notice it. It was worse at night when she lied down in bed, and she started propping herself up with pillows so that she wouldn't cough as much.

One night, about a week before her appointment, we were lying quietly in bed and she whispered almost to herself, "I can feel it burning inside my body again." By the way that her voice was shaking, I could tell that she was really scared. It scared me too

85

because she had come to know her body. The last time she had this same feeling she was very right. Still, I refused to believe that the cow could return so quickly. I whispered back to her, "It's just all those phlegm balls rolling around in your lungs. Just give it a couple of those hearty hacks like your dad does in the morning and you will get rid of that crud." There was no response except for a disgusted cough in my general direction.

It was time for Lisa's appointment, and as usual I took off work, picked her up at home, and we drove together to meet the doctor. Sitting in the oncology waiting room was always very depressing. Many of the people there were either taking treatments or were waiting for the dreaded test results. Not once had I ever seen anyone give anyone else a high five in this place. The routine we knew all too well, and it always involved waiting. Waiting for blood to be drawn, waiting for the results, waiting for the doctor to show up, waiting for time to pass. We had been brainwashed by the cow into accepting delays and had developed a kind of numb patience.

The 'ist' guy came in with his usual blunt sarcasm, which I found kind of refreshing but Lisa had no tolerance for. She did not want to laugh or smile, she just wanted to get in and get out. He did his usual thumping, poking and prodding ritual on her neck, back and chest and then asked, "How have you been feeling?"

"I feel fine," and she paused as if unsure whether to

continue. She got a running start and tried again. "I feel fine except I've had this runny nose and a little cough."

"Cough," he said suspiciously with raised eyebrows. "We had better do an x-ray just as a precaution."

Lisa gave no reaction as if she knew that this was going to happen, and I suspect she did. The nurse led her off for some pictures. When Lisa came back we put our numb patience to a test as we waited silently for the pictures to be developed.

The 'ist' returned without the nurse and with his dry candor delivered the verdict like the head juror of a murder trial, "You are coughing because your lungs are covered with cancer."

Her face dropped to the floor along with my heart. "Am I going to die," Lisa asked already knowing the answer.

"Yes."

She shrunk further into her chair, "How much time do I have?"

"If you do nothing you might have six months," he stated without hesitation as if this was a standard answer quoted to people in Lisa's condition. Then I saw Lisa crawl into her shell and the rest of the conversation was between the doctor and I. "Do you want to try more chemotherapy?"

"What would you do," I asked.

"Take the chemo and pray for a miracle."

I looked at Lisa and she shrugged her slumping shoulders,

as in her mind she didn't have another choice. I took that as a yes. "When do we start?"

"Tomorrow morning if you want." Then we went home to lay this bombshell on her parents.

The chemotherapy did some good the first month but that was it. Then her body started to deteriorate very rapidly as her lungs started to drown in the fluid generated from the cancer cells. We knew that now was the time to tell the kids that their mom was going to die. Lisa felt very strongly about telling the kids by herself, so she gave them the "mommy's going to die" speech while I was at work. She did not tell me much about how the talk went other than that Samantha told her that she was not scared because her dad had been taking care of them for a long time and would do a good job.

Our kids had been amazing throughout this whole ordeal. Some of the credit for their success should go to Lisa and I, as we made a conscious effort to be up front and honest with them from the very beginning. We explained cancer, chemotherapy, and the hair loss. We told them cancer was a very bad disease that people die from, and that the doctors were doing their best to make their mom better. When Lisa was quarantined in the hospital for five weeks for the stem cell transplant I drew the kids a picture of her room so they could visualize where she was. The hospital also let us borrow a video telephone for one week so we could talk to and see her on the phone. Each night we gathered around the little screen like it was family TV night. When Lisa finally got home from the hospital and had to wear those hospital masks all the time, I wrote the kids a short story that explained why it was so important to keep germs out of her lungs. Samantha took the story to school for her first grade teacher to read to her class, which made Sam feel special and stopped all the kids on the bus from making fun of her masked mom.

Probably the most important thing we did for the kids was to surround them with people that loved them, which made them feel safe. They never had to worry about being cared for. Sometimes they got sad about what was happening to their mom but they never appeared to be scared or worried about what would happen to them.

Lisa's mission for the rest of her life was quite clear: Save the children. She was going to prepare the kids, our family, and the entire city if necessary, to make sure everyone and everything was in place before her departure. She made sure their shots were up to date, bedrooms were painted, closets arranged, car pools established, day care lined up, and so on. By far the most important thing to her was getting the school situation for Samantha and Emily straightened out. The city we lived in had a mandatory lottery based on birth date. If our kid's birth date was drawn out of the magic hat, they would get bused to the magnet school (which was located in a section of town known for gang related activity) instead of taking the short and safe bus ride to the school in our neighborhood. "Did you check the paper for the lottery dates yet?" Lisa asked as she rolled the paper tightly in her hands.

"No, not yet," but I could tell that she had. "Let me guess. One of their birth dates got picked."

"Nope, both of them were picked," she snapped in disgust. "This is the stupidest damn system. I thought when we moved from the East we got away from busing."

"Maybe we can apply for special consideration or some kind of hardship. I'm sure it happens every year."

"If it hasn't ever happened before, this will definitely be the first." Then she flung the paper at me and left the room muttering.

"In this corner wearing a combination of old rules and regulations is The Public School System. In the other corner, the challenger, a dying mother with four children and dressed in solid motherhood, our very own Lisa."

The school system didn't stand a chance. If this had been a pay-per-view fight, all those who paid to watch would have been disappointed because it was a first round knockout and she didn't even have to throw a punch. The reason for the short fight was that a really nice thing happened on the way to Madison Square Garden; something that made me feel good about people again. The principal from our then-current school knew of Lisa's health condition, and knew that there were a lot of good reasons that our kids needed to be at a school close to home. She actually took the time to look up Samantha's and Emily's birth dates and then checked the paper to see if they were listed. As soon as she saw their dates in the paper she made a couple of phone calls and the next thing we knew we received a letter in the mail confirming their enrollment in the school we had wanted. The rest of our kids would now automatically follow their siblings and Lisa did not have to worry about their school situation anymore.

As for me, I felt like I was the dummy in a military camp that was used for bayonet practice. Lisa wanted me to know how she did everything, and she wanted me to do them exactly the same way. The laundry was a major concern. She cringed when she watched me sort my own laundry into two piles, a sweaty stuff pile and a non-sweaty stuff pile. "Whose are these," she asked as she held up a pair of panties with cute little teddy bears.

"Emily's?"

"Wrong, they are Samantha's. How about these?"

I just shrugged my shoulders in defeat. Then I held up a pair of underwear with a Red Power Ranger in the back and a strategically placed yellow stain in the front. "These are too small to be mine so they must be Ben's," I said soliciting a smile from Lisa. Apparently, there also was a certain way to put laundry into the washer, which had something to do with whether the detergent went in before or after the clothes. I tried to keep up, but I was still lost from the sorting lesson. Making school lunches was another eye opening experience. Crust on, crust off, vanilla pudding, chocolate pudding, each kid had preferences that had been in front of my face for years, but I never had taken the time to notice. I never had to before. There was a list of things a mile long which would have been overwhelming on its own had there been time to actually worry about it. As it was, between my work and her failing health I was already treading pretty low in the water.

The kids seemed to take every major change in their mom's health in stride. Their protective bubbles had been burst a while ago and it appeared that nothing could shock them. Whenever possible we gave them advanced warning as to any new developments. The hair loss from the chemo was old hat for them, even for Gaven who was only three. "Hey kids, your mom's hair is going to start falling out next week," or "She won't be able to hug you for awhile because the doctor cut off the breast that had cancer and it is going to hurt her for a long time." At one point the fluid in her lungs had built up so fast that her heart had a hard time beating and she had to be rushed by ambulance to the hospital for emergency surgery. "Kids, your mom got sick and had to go to the hospital last night."

"What's wrong with her? Is it the cancer?" they asked in

concert.

"Yes, the fluid made by the cancer cells was all around her heart and it made it real hard for it to beat and pump blood to the rest of her body."

"Did the doctors fix her?" asked Ben.

"They tried. They cut a small window in this bag that goes around her heart so the liquid can get out," I explained. They looked confused so I tested my art skills and drew them a picture. It seemed to help.

"Then where does the fluid go?"

"You guys sure do ask a lot of really good questions."

They seemed to understand or were at least comforted simply because I took the time to try to explain it to them. Just knowing that there was an explanation seemed to help.

Following her surgery Lisa was stuck in the hospital for a couple of weeks, and the kids were excited about visiting Mom because the nurses usually gave them ice cream. They made get well cards and took turns sitting with her on her hospital bed. Emily, who was six, got a little nervous because she was afraid she might accidentally pull on one of the tubes connected to her mom's arm and neck. With all of us crammed into a small hospital room, things were a bit nerve-racking, so we never stayed long. Lisa hated being in the hospital, mainly because she couldn't spend time with her kids. Because Kansas is so flat, we could see the hospital from the highway and the kids would wave and yell as we were coming and going, "That's where our mom is!" How come they were always capable of seeing something good in almost every rotten situation? Why do we have to lose that mentality when we grow older?

Lisa's fear of dying in the hospital made her quite adamant about going home. "After I get home I don't want to be fixed or patched up anymore. If something else goes wrong just let me die, okay?"

I just nodded that I understood, but it would not be an easy request for me to fulfill.

When we were ready to leave the hospital, she tried to stand up and walk, and fell back into her bed in severe pain. The cancer had spread to her hip and she could no longer support herself. She came home confined to a wheelchair and pissed off at the world. The kids had a hard time understanding why she went into the hospital to get fixed and came home seemingly more broken than before. It was, however, somewhat gratifying for the children to be able to push her from one room to another. But I think it was torture for Lisa, as she had to accept the fact that she would never walk again. The circumstances were getting grimmer but we persisted with telling the kids everything in as much detail as they could understand, which was quite a lot considering their ages.

Not only did she come home in a wheelchair, but also

during those two weeks in the hospital the cancer in her lungs had progressed to the point that she needed oxygen. We decided that the time had come to hire hospice care. Hospice was covered by our insurance only if in the doctor's opinion she had less than six months to live. He did not hesitate to sign the appropriate form. During my fat, dumb and happy life I had never heard of hospice until my friend Bruce from work mentioned it in reference to his grandmother. Now they were in my house, putting a note on our refrigerator door signed by our doctor that says 'Do Not Resuscitate.' This was the legal document needed so that the doctors and nurses would not try to save her life anymore. That was fun to look at every time we needed to get the milk. They also brought in a hospital-style bed, a port-a-potty, an oxygen machine, and a nurse. I had to scoot our bed over against the wall to make room for her new bed. We never slept in the same bed together again.

The kids thought all these new gadgets were kind of cool. They liked pushing the buttons on the remote control bed, and zipping around in the hot rod wheelchair. They also enjoyed watching the gauges and lights on the oxygen machine, which sounded like Darth Vader and looked like R2D2. They were amazed at the oxygen tube that Lisa used which was long enough to run the entire length of the house. They still played around her as if nothing were wrong. She liked seeing them run by and hearing them laugh but she was still the boss and would on occasion bark out a command to remind them of that fact. At night they would come down to her bed to rub her head, give her a hug and say good night. I wondered, as they lay in their beds at night, if they thought about how sick their mom was. They had to have wished that their mom could run and play with them, or take them shopping at the mall, watch their dives at the pool, or just come upstairs to tuck them in. How many nights she cried because she couldn't.

Lisa's pain started to get very intense, and she was given a prescription for morphine. When I went to the drug store, the pharmacist knew exactly why I needed these drugs and gave me a nod of understanding. Her pain was constant and rapidly intensifying which made it impossible to keep up with, so the hospice nurse hooked her up with a morphine pump. This machine, which hung at her side like a Sony Walkman, would give her a programmed dose on regular intervals. If the pain got too intense she could push a magic button that would give her an extra shot.

Morphine is a wicked drug. She couldn't live without it, but living with it and its side effects was unbearable to her. She hallucinated often, talking to imaginary people and not really knowing what she was saying. Much of the time she did not know who the kids or I were. It was during one of these moments that I first saw the kids look at her like she was a freak. It was a painful thing to watch. Sometimes she would start yelling loud enough that the kids could hear her from the other room. One time Ben, who was four, was cruising through the house and he heard her yell something that sounded like "Jumanji." Ben stopped running for a second, looked over at me, rolled his eyes and with a sad grin said, "There's that crazy Mom of mine." Then he was off running again. The worst of it was that Lisa, the mom, the person, was still in there somewhere and often would know that she was talking gibberish but still couldn't stop doing it. She would get angry and vow to cut back on the morphine. Dealing with the pain had to be better than being this crazy person who was scaring her own kids. Then the pain would creep up to the screaming point, and it would be back to pushing the magic button. During a lucid moment, before the drugs reclaimed their control, she started crying loudly. I ran into the bedroom, "What's wrong. Are you in a lot of pain?"

"It's not too bad yet," she claimed as tears rolled down her cheeks. "But it's coming and I can't do it without the drugs. I thought I could, but it hurts too much and now I am going to be a crazy, babbling drug addict for what's left of my life, and that's what the kids are going to remember about me."

"The kids know that isn't you. They know it's the medicine and cancer making you this way. They will remember you as you were. I'll make sure of that, I promise." She winced and pushed the button for more morphine.

Even though their mom considered herself somewhat of a monster, the kids refused to be swayed. One of the most horrible yet beautiful things happened on Samantha's eighth birthday. We had a party for her at our house, and Lisa's mom came over to help out. About the time the other kids arrived Lisa was doped up and sleeping very soundly. "Do you think I should try to wake her up for the party," I asked Lisa's mom.

"I don't know. It's hard to tell how she is going to be. I would hate for her to miss Samantha's birthday."

"Yeah, me too, but it would be hard on Samantha if she started talking nonsense or screaming in front of all of her friends. She is pretty out of it right now. I think I will let her sleep for a while and try to wake her up a little later," I said trying to convince myself that was the right thing to do.

Well, as decisions like these go, just as Samantha was unwrapping this special nightgown that her mom had ordered for her months in advance just in case she wasn't around anymore, Lisa woke up. She didn't just open her eyes and start looking around the room like she had just pecked her way through an eggshell, she woke with an eerie kind of instant clarity. She knew exactly what was going on. "How could you not wake me for the last birthday that I will ever have a chance to see," she screamed angrily. God we felt horrible. Lisa's mom was visibly crushed. We got Lisa out of bed and wheeled her into the room where the party was and parked her right next to Sam. Samantha gave her a big hug, and was thrilled that her mom could join her for her party. "Thanks so much for the nightgown, it's just what I wanted." Then Sam went around the room introducing her Mom to all of her friends. Sam was great and saved the party with the nonchalant way she accepted her mother's condition. It put all of us at ease. Sam knew that her mom was not the cancer and not the morphine; for her it was like "The Emperor's New Clothes," only in reverse. The other kids stared at Lisa for a moment and then went on about their business. Once again I had underestimated the minds and hearts of our children. Never in a million years would Samantha ever be embarrassed on account of her mom. I also should have known that it would take a lot more than a little morphine and a cancer-ridden body to keep Lisa from Samantha's party. My decision to protect everyone from embarrassment backfired, and maybe it was really me who I was trying to protect all along. After the party, Lisa's mom was still shaken as she felt as though she had let her daughter down. She apologized deeply and then left for home in tears.

Day in and day out I was learning so much about what love and life were truly about just from watching how Lisa and our children carried on. It's unfortunate how the world corrupts that innocent love and innate wisdom to the point that it's lost in us. What I was finding out was that this child-like ability to love was still there locked up just waiting to be released. This kind of love is not a thought in your head or words that fall way too casually out of your mouth, but it's a feeling down deep in your gut. My kids were the key, and it took this tragedy to bring this realization to light. It was like the gas furnace kicking on that first frosty fall morning. Smelling the heat first, giving a sense of the warmth soon to follow. Then as the heat pushes the cold into the corners and cracks, a tingle runs up your spine like the mercury in the thermometer. It's the feeling of love that generates a mother's or a child's warmth, not the words. Lisa's furnace was cranked up as high as it would go and she kept us all warm for as long as she could.

Months earlier, Lisa and I had started to have one of those fun discussions about whether she should be buried of cremated. We tried to think which would be easiest for the kids, but we never came to a consensus and never had the chance to get back to it. By the time I was faced with having to figure this out, Lisa was pretty much incoherent. It was left up to me to decide. My theory when it came to the kids was when in doubt, just ask them. So one Saturday afternoon I interrupted a game of baseball down in our basement. "It's time for a family meeting."

"Oh man, can I bat first?" whined Ben with a bat in his hands.

"This won't take long but it is very important," as I gestured everyone over to the couch. "Does anyone know what it means for someone to be cremated?"

Samantha raised her hand, "I've heard of it but I can't remember what it is. Does it happen to dead people?"

"Yes it does. When people die they are either put in a big box called a casket and buried under the ground, or they can be cremated. When someone is cremated they put the body in a real hot fire until it turns to ashes. Kind of like a how a log in a fireplace turns to ashes. Then the ashes are put in a big jar called an urn and given to the dead person's family."

"What does the family do with the ashes?"

"They can keep the urn in the house just to have around or take the ashes and spread them around a pretty garden or throw them up into the wind. Whatever they want to do. What should we do if your mom dies?"

"The fire would hurt, I don't want my mommy burned," piped in Gaven.

"Ya, let's bury her in a cemetery, in one of those caskets," suggested Samantha as everyone shouted their approval.

"Okay, that's what we will do. See that wasn't so bad. Aren't I a fun dad to have around? Next week's family meeting we will discuss the various methods of embalming." They looked at me like I was crazy. "All right, let's Play Ball!"

As it became obvious that the end was near, the kids and I had many talks about what would happen to their mom after she died. I'm not the kind of guy to preach or push religion on anyone, but we did make our kids go to Sunday school which is where they learned about angels. They learned that angels are good and that they watch over us. Church is worth its weight in gold if for no other reason than to give your kids something to hang this death hat on. Later in life, when they are old enough to figure out what they want to believe in, they would be free to decide what place church would have in their lives. But for now it comforted them and me so much to know that their mom would be this beautiful angel who checked in on them at night.

After I told my new boss that my wife's cancer was back and that I would be gone from work now and then, she really left me alone. In fact, everyone in my group treated me as if I really wasn't there. It was like being a shadow. I could pass right down the center aisle creating nothing more than a whisper. As before, I ended up with no real assignments. My rubber ball of a career had very few bounces left in it at that point.

As they had in Philadelphia, the kids started to resent the way that their grandparents were treating them. In other words, their grandparents were treating them as if they were their own kids and this was not always well received. Grandparents aren't usually the ones to tell the grandkids to clean their room and that they can't have another snack. It's traditionally quite the opposite, with the grandparents swooping in with treats and presents for a quick dose of spoiling. Sadly, their grandparents were not allowed to practice this tradition, at least at that time. Some nights Ben would ask me if Grandpa would be coming over again in the morning, and after I told him yes, he would act disappointed. I wished it could be different. No one liked this arrangement, but in tough times you just do the best you can and hope somewhere down the road it gets better.

One day, as I came home for lunch to check on Lisa and to meet with the nurse, there was a new and important development in Lisa's condition. Her heart, which for the past month had been racing at an unbelievable rate of about 160 beats per minute had suddenly slowed way down and was decreasing by the hour. Her face had relaxed. Before it had been so anguished that her forehead was permanently scrunched up and her upper lip was stretched tight across her teeth. Somewhere inside she had finally conceded that the cow was going to win this battle here on earth. Following this acceptance was an inner peace, which was apparent to us as we watched her in her coma-like sleep. By the time the kids were ready for bed her heart rate had dropped to about nine beats a minute and there was a good chance that she wasn't going to make it through the night. After the kids each hugged and kissed their mom good night I took them all up to Samantha's bedroom for a little chat. This was not going to be the kind of chat that you would want to have with your child anytime, let alone just before they were going to bed, but it had to happen. "Hey guys, everyone up on Samantha's bed. We need to have a quick family meeting."

"Again?" fussed a tired Emily.

"Yes, again." They all piled on Sam's bed, sensing I was going to say something important as they had grown accustomed to these family meetings. "There is a real good chance that your mom will die sometime tonight." They all stared at me with mouths and eyes wide open. "If she does would you like me to wake you so you can say good-bye to her?"

They all nodded 'yes' with their tired, confused little heads, and just as I was about to carry them off to each of their beds Lisa's dad hollered up the stairs that I had better get down there. So I left the kids all sitting on Sam's bed wondering who knows what, and ran down to Lisa's room where I found everyone standing around her bed watching her struggle to take a breath. It truly couldn't have been more than a minute or two before she took in one last breath and held it, this last bittersweet taste of a life that had ended so prematurely.

Who Saved Who

       I had never been to a funeral. I had never known anyone who had died.   Never in my wildest dreams or nightmares did I imagine that I would actually watch someone die right before my eyes, let alone my thirty-six year old wife.

       For months this nightmare had been building up to this inevitable moment and then as quick as a simple breath it was over. I can't help but think of a roller coaster as it slowly clinks and clanks up that first and biggest hill, when it seems like you will never reach the top. Finally, you're at the summit and the roller coaster stops for a suspense-filled pause. The cars are resting directly beneath the sign which reads "The Point of No Return" and it's true, there really is no way out. Ready or not here it goes. Then with a slight jerk it starts down, dropping so fast that you want to scream but you can't, you want to let go and raise your hands high above your head but you remain white-knuckled to the safety bar. Your lungs forget how to exhale and your heart wants to stop but instead it beats wildly (or maybe that's backwards). All that's around you is a blur, voices no longer have an owner, and like an uncontrollable dream, thoughts and visions flash in front of you. You're blasted with a rush of mixed up sensations, but before you have a chance to get your bearings the car hits the brakes and the faces with their voices come back into focus.

Her parents, my parents, her brother-in-law, her sister and I just stood silently at Lisa's bedside for a moment. Her sister broke out of the trance and checked Lisa's pulse and noted the time. We all took turns saying good-bye. I kissed her forehead and pressed my cheek against hers. It was difficult for me to digest, but there was no time for me now as I jumped back into the front seat of the roller coaster and clinked my way back upstairs to break the news to the kids.

They were all exactly where I had left them right beneath the "point of no return" sign. "Your mom just died," I said quietly as I gave the roller coaster a push. At first I don't think they believed me because it happened so quickly after our talk. Samantha gave out a nervous little laugh, obviously not knowing how to act in this situation. Emily started to cry and Ben stomped around and kicked at the bed. Little Gaven, who was just three years old, looked to her big sister to see what she was supposed to do and forced out a similar laugh. Then I scooped up Ben and Gaven in my arms, and with Samantha and Emily clutching on to my legs we rode the roller coaster breathlessly down the stairs, somehow without flying off the tracks. Then the roller coaster hit the brakes and one by one the kids stopped at her bedside, hugged her neck, kissed her bald head, and said farewell to their mother. Just then Ben went shooting out of the room, through the house, and out the back door. I chased after him to see if he was all right, but by the time I caught up to him he was already heading back in. "What were you doing outside, Ben?"

"I wanted to see if I could see Mom's spirit rising to heaven, but I must have been too late," he said as he scuffed his foot at the floor.

"Your Mom flew up to heaven as fast as she could so she could become an angel and start watching over you as soon as possible," I reassured Ben as I gave him a big hug.

"Is she with other angels?"

"Definitely. Because your mom was so special the other angels were all waiting to take care of her. Now let's get something to drink."

The kids, as expected, were wound up tight. To them, in an unnatural way, this was almost like a party. Pastor George came over and he gathered everyone around Lisa where we held hands as he said a prayer, which I wish I could remember. I don't think I was even listening; there was too much noise in my head. Then I put the kids to bed. They all wanted to sleep in the same room, which sounded reasonable to me. Before Lisa's stem cell transplant she wrote them each a special note to keep under their pillows while she was gone. As I tucked the kids in I read their special letter to each of them. It was as if their mom was tucking them in bed. Then Ben and Samantha doubled up in Emily and Gaven's room and fell asleep rather easily, as they were emotionally and physically wiped out from the wild roller coaster ride.

After the people from the mortuary took Lisa's body away in some kind of a body bag, the adults hung around in the kitchen for awhile longer, and with no disrespect to Lisa, tried to make small talk. It was kind of like taking a time out, as we all needed to take a breather. Finally, everyone reached that point of exhaustive understanding and decided it was time to get some rest. We all knew there would be plenty of things to do in the days ahead.

Then suddenly it was quiet. There was a hush over the house that hadn't been there for months. Even the constant humming of R2D2, the 24-hour oxygen machine was silent. I laid down in my bed, next to the now empty mechanical bed, and got the best night's sleep I'd had in a real long time.

Planning for the memorial service and funeral was like planning a shotgun wedding. Not that I have ever been involved in a shotgun wedding, but I've heard stories. Scheduling the pastor, the church, ordering food, notifying friends and relatives, deciding on flowers, buying a casket, writing sermons for the memorial and funeral service, picking the right music, arranging places to stay for out of town guests. It was all done in a matter of hours.

Take my advice, if you know a loved one is going to die and if you have time to plan the services in advance, don't wait like we did until after the fact. The only things Lisa told me were that she wanted the memorial service to be for the kids, and that she did not want me wasting a lot of money burying her. Her request that I not spend a lot of money to bury her came in handy when I was being pressured by the casket salesman to buy the super deluxe nuclear resistant titanium alloyed box with a 10,000 year rust proof guarantee and a $10,000,000 price tag. The thing looked like a torpedo or something that would send her back to the future. All I had to keep telling the guy was that my wife wanted the least expensive casket and in the end he had a hard time arguing with the wishes of the deceased.

One of the hardest things was deciding what day to have the funeral. The tricky part about this was that Lisa died on the Friday of Labor Day weekend and the following Tuesday was the first day of school. We couldn't have it on the Monday holiday because there were bound to be a lot of people on vacation. Tuesday would have been a good day but I wasn't sure how to handle the first day of school for Samantha and Emily. Lisa and many others had worked so hard to get them into a particular school and I knew that she had really wanted to live long enough to see them get on that bus on the first day. Because the memorial service really was to be for the kids, it made sense that they have a voice in the matter. "Hey Samantha and Emily, come here for a second I need to ask you guys something."

They came running up the basement stairs sounding like a herd of horses. "What is it Dad," they asked as they practically fell over each other.

"Would you guys rather that your mom's funeral be on Tuesday, which is the first day of school, or the day after on Wednesday?"

"I don't want to miss the first day of school," pleaded Samantha.

"Me neither," agreed Emily.

"Really, are you guys sure? The first day of school could be kind of tough."

"We're sure. The first day is the most important one. You learn where the bathrooms are, what time you eat lunch, who you sit by in class and all that stuff," Samantha said like a seasoned veteran.

"Yeah and we have never ridden a bus before and we can't miss the first day," added Emily.

"Thanks, you helped me make a very important decision. The funeral will be on Wednesday," I declared to the delight of the girls.

My worry had been that they would be emotionally unable to go to school and deal with those situations where a teacher or a student asks about their mom. I called the principal, with whom I had been in close contact over the last few weeks, and let her know what had happened so that she could notify their teachers. The kids handled the decisions about school very maturely, and once again totally defused a situation over which I had lost many healthy hairs. They made these tough decisions not so tough. All I had to do was ask them, as things were very clear in their young, uncluttered minds. The biggest mistake I could have made would have been to underestimate my kids and not give them the opportunity to express their opinions. By participating in the decisions that affected them, they felt that they were important.

A group of about twelve family members met at my house on Saturday afternoon to hurriedly plan the services. Whenever there was a decision that we could not reach by consensus, all eyes turned to me to make the final decision. It was the first time in my life that a room full of very smart and talented people wanted me to make the important decisions. This made me very nervous at first, but once I realized the magnitude of this responsibility I forgot about my insecurities, and my thoughts and opinions started coming to me clearly. I kept focused on the theme, which was to keep it very simple and to make it for the kids.

My success handling this situation altered a trait of mine, which I had always viewed as a flaw. In group situations I never had the confidence to voice my opinions for fear of looking dumb. I can remember an incident in my early childhood that I believe could have been a major factor in making me this way. When I was about seven, my brothers and I and the rest of the neighborhood boys were bored one summer afternoon and were doing stupid things on our bikes. Big surprise. We were trying to see who could go the furthest on our bikes down this extremely bumpy drainage ditch with our feet up in the air. The trick was to get a lot of speed so as to produce enough momentum to make it over the first big bump. Boys can be pretty goofy all by themselves, but to make matters worse there were a couple of the neighborhood girls sitting on the porch pretending not to be watching. That's all the audience I needed. I was going to show those girls that I was the coolest and proceeded to get my bike moving faster than anyone else. I hit that first bump so hard that it threw me forward, off my seat, where I landed straddling the handlebars. Then I flipped over the front of the bike, landing flat on my back. If getting my breath knocked out of me and having my testicles smashed weren't bad enough, as I picked myself up off the ground I heard those girls laughing. I just knew they were laughing at me, and as I was running up the hill with one hand on my crotch and the other on my ribs I kept getting madder and madder. When I reached the porch I yelled at those girls something intelligent like "If you think it's so funny I would like to see you try it!"

"Try what?" they snapped. "We weren't laughing at you and if you think we were even watching you, you're crazy". Then they did start laughing at me, and the other guys who had barely enough time to stop laughing from my wipe out started up again as they enjoyed watching me make a big fool out of myself. From that moment I had subconsciously decided that unless I was dead certain that I knew what I was talking about I would keep my mouth shut.

The day before their mom's funeral, Samantha and Emily slung backpacks over their shoulders and climbed onto the school bus for the first day of school. It was quite a scene as all four of their grandparents, their aunt and uncle, their little brother Ben and sister Gaven, their dog and me all escorted them to the bus stop. They loved the attention and were very excited. Of course what was missing in this picture was their mom, whose long-range goal had been to live long enough to see this moment. It's amazing how small and simple our lives are when you really boil it down. I had offered to drive them to school but they had never ridden a school bus before and insisted on the experience. As the bus pulled away with them smiling and waving out the window, I was so proud of their resilience and unforced natural strength. It gave all of us who were there a huge shot in the arm. We needed it because the world keeps spinning fast even though our little roller coaster was taking one of those suspense-filled pauses at the top of the hill.

The days leading up to the memorial service were a blur with friends and family working together in a surprisingly organized and calm fashion. Pastor George was taking care of putting together the service. He would be quoting from a couple of books that he had given to my children. He thought it would be comforting if they heard something familiar. Lisa's mom walked up to me and handed me two journals. "Have you read these yet?"

"What are they?" I asked without opening them.

"They are a couple of journals that Lisa actually wrote some things in," she said in a surprised tone.

"That's kind of hard to believe. She always told me she hated journals and got perturbed when all her friends kept sending them to her for gifts."

"I know it. Well, she didn't write much, but when you get a moment you really should read through them," she repeated.

There was no time to read them but I ran them to George at the church and told him he should feel free to use anything in those journals that would be appropriate for the service, which was less than 24 hours away.

My sisters-in-law scrambled around looking for pictures of Lisa, young and old, to make a Lisa story board. They found Lisa's famous Xerox box filled with hundreds of loosely stacked pictures which had always been intended for photo albums that never happened. I stood for a moment and watched as they hurriedly sifted through all the pictures. The memories each photo brought to life made me both happy and sad.

Cradling the hug shaped shoebox of photographs,
Her mother lying face up, flipped over, turned to the side.
Open the box yesterday and she is full of laughs,
Peaks beneath the lid today and she cried.

No different really than the ashes in the urn,
Memories of her remains all intertwined.
Close your eyes and the pictures return,
A shoe box of photographs burned into her mind.

It took some time but they were able to make two picture storyboards that started with her as a baby and ended with her having babies. These they framed and placed on easels in the entrance to the church. One of Lisa's best friends had agreed to sing at the service. We picked the songs in a hurry. One of them was a song that Lisa's mom liked to listen to when Lisa was calm and sleeping. Lisa's mom also had saved a bunch of pictures that the kids had drawn and colored over the past couple of years for their mom. These drawings were taped to an old door and placed up by the altar. I wasn't sure what George had intended to do in the service, but I knew that the kids would recognize their own handy-work.

In my opinion, the most meaningful thing that occurred (which was unknown to almost everyone) was that Samantha, with the help of Lisa's sister, actually picked out the dress and jewelry that her mom was going to be buried in. "Samantha, could you help me pick out some clothes for your mom to be buried in. We want her to look pretty and I thought you might know what she liked to wear," said her aunt as they walked into her mom's closet.

"What is she wearing now?" Samantha asked a bit con-fused.

"She still has on the pajamas she was wearing the night she died, so we thought she would like to have a change of clothes. Did she have a favorite dress," she asked as she flipped through the hangers.

"I'm not sure which one was her favorite but I always thought she looked the prettiest in this one," Sam said as she grabbed for the bright orange and yellow striped dress.

"Oh yes," said her aunt, "This was one of her favorites and it is very colorful. It will be perfect. Good choice Samantha."

Samantha smiled proudly, "Can we pick out some ear-rings too?"

The kids all had a good visual image of their mom, lying peacefully in a comfy coffin wearing her orange dress. This would not have been possible if we had decided to have her cremated.

The morning of the service finally arrived and I had plenty of help getting the kids dressed. There were dresses for the girls, and ties and sport coats for us boys. We actually got to the church on time. The kids were quiet and somewhat apprehensive, as they really had no idea what to expect. Neither did I.

We waited in the church's parlor until most of the guests had arrived. We were then ushered in as inconspicuously as possible from the side and took our place in the front row. As I walked in I could sense that all eyes were on the kids and me. I could see out of the corner of my eye that the place was full, but I didn't dare make direct eye contact with anyone because no one likes to see a superhero cry, especially my kids. This was the ultimate not crying test. If I made it through this day without shedding a tear then it would prove that my tear ducts had dried up years ago.

I felt as though I was the magic feather that Dumbo held in his trunk to make him believe that he could do the impossible and fly. There these four young children stood, with the spotlight directly on them as they were about to be asked to go up on stage at their own mother's funeral. If I were to have a mental meltdown the magic feather would slip out of their tiny little fingers and they surely would have fallen. Then I realized that I was the one who was struggling to maintain my composure and that they were the feathers and I was Dumbo. In the end we held on to each other and that's what got us through.

Lisa's friend Suzy asked the kids to come up front and sit on the steps as she sang a song. This was pure entertainment for them and they loved it. Then George called them over one at a time to the old door with all of their artwork stuck to it and asked them various questions about these pictures. Which ones were theirs, what or who was it a picture of, why they drew it, and so on. Samantha took great pleasure in speaking into the microphone and telling the audience about her pictures. Emily, on the other hand, was rather shy and was about to freeze up, until George asked her which of the drawings were hers. She started pointing to each of her drawings and realized that most of them on the door were hers. George was impressed, "Wow Emily, are these really all your drawings?"

"Yes," she eeked.

"You are quite a good artist. I bet your mom really enjoyed getting these from you."

That gave Emily the confidence boost she needed as she started to describe in detail what each drawing was and why she drew it. She began to ramble and George almost had to cut her off. She walked back to her seat feeling quite good about herself.

Ben and Gaven were both a bit overwhelmed as they grunted and mumbled their answers to George's questions.

Later in the service George started quoting passages from Lisa's journals, which of course were new to me since I hadn't read them. But what he read were little pieces of advice she had written for her kids. She told the girls how old they should be before they should have their ears pierced, and she told Ben not to play football because she thought it was too violent. George had a good way of talking directly to each of the children and made it kind of humorous. "Ben," George said looking directly at him, "If you ever want to play football, just come and talk to me and we will see if we can work something out." The kids all laughed and felt very special, and they'll never forget their mom's advice. Of course they won't necessarily listen. If I were smart I would forge some entries in that journal like, "no dating until you are 21 and have moved out of your dad's house," and, "Get a job so you can buy your own clothes." I could keep adding to the journal to cover other difficult situations that were sure to pop up over the years to come. Then I would just have to pull out the magic book and say, "Your mom says right here that you can't get a tattoo."

Throughout the entire service the kids kept their poise, with the exception of Gaven's crawling around on my lap and grabbing on to my neck (which was actually a good distraction for me). They pulled me through the service. I was not ready to deal with the emotions of Lisa's death, nor did I have the time.

I stood in the parlor after the memorial service in somewhat of a receiving line, allowing friends and relatives to hug me and tell me how sorry they were and if I ever needed anything and so on. One friend of mine from work came through the line with his wife, and when he saw me he just broke down and started bawling. They had three young children of their own and it saddened him to think of my children or theirs without a mother. A year later they started having marital problems and his wife moved out. It makes me wonder which is harder on kids, having a parent die or living through a divorce. I'm sure the 'ist' people have written books on the subject.

After all the people finally cleared out, there was a luncheon for family members down in the basement of the church. It was impossible to get a moment to sit and eat. There was always one more person who wanted to say something. I really wasn't hungry but I forced down a sandwich on the run because the day was just beginning. We still had to drive a hundred miles to the cemetery for the funeral service, which basically was closed to non-family members.

The cemetery sat on top of a hill overlooking a lake out in the middle of nowhere. This cemetery was close to the small towns where Lisa's mom and dad grew up, and was the place where many of their family members were buried. The children thought it was neat that their mom was going to be buried next to her grandparents, aunts, uncles and possibly her own parents.

It was sunny and hot on top of that hill and I started to sweat as we waited for everyone to make their way to this out-of-the-way place. Of course the only people that had trouble finding it were my parents. They missed a turn, so I had to sweat wondering where in the hell they could be. The kids were miserable and everyone was just wandering around the cemetery. George walked up to me, "What do you want to do?"

"Give it five more minutes and then start the ceremony whether they are here or not."

I measured the minutes by counting the beads of sweat roll off my nose. Fortunately, to everyone's relief, with about one minute (or ten drips) to spare they came tearing up the road and we were ready to start.

The casket was resting under a small tent and was covered with long stem roses. Attached to one of the handles were four helium-filled balloons, one for each kid. It was obvious that George intended to have the children let their balloons loose sometime during the ceremony.

While we were waiting for my parents to show, Emily's balloon blew into the roses and popped. There is no doubt in my mind that I had some kind of a small stroke. Of all the kids, Emily seemed to be taking this day the hardest. She would have been the last one that I thought could handle something like that. But before either of us had a chance to get upset, Samantha came up with a

121

solution, "That's okay Emily, we can all hang onto the balloons and let them go at the same time." Emily was noticeably relieved as she accepted this solution with an ever so slight smile, which was huge for her. When the time came to let go of the balloons, the four of them stood in a huddle like a basketball team just before the start of a game. Then on the count of three they let loose of the strings at the top of their reach and they left their arms raised to the sky like statues. We all watched the different colored balloons get caught in that reliable Kansas breeze and head up and out over the lake. Everyone was silent until the balloons were out of sight.

The letting go of balloons became a standard ritual for any occasion related to their mom. Her birthday, her death day, and Mother's day were all balloon events. Now, no matter what the occasion, whenever any of them got a balloon, they'd always let it go thinking that their mom would catch it and use it to keep her afloat up in heaven.

After the service everyone piled into their cars and headed back to our house for pizza, horseshoes and beer. It had been a long, emotional day and I don't believe I have ever had a better tasting, more deserved beer in my life.

The next morning most of the out of town family members bolted for home, and there I was. I took three weeks off from work and spent my days doing kid related tasks. Grocery shopping, laundry, cooking meals, teacher conferences, and art class registrations. I was doing all those things that Lisa was afraid wouldn't happen. I even got myself connected into the mommy network and found some good day care for Ben and Gaven, arranged carpools and play dates with other kids, and got Sam and Emily enrolled in the after-school program. Everything sort of fell into place. Don't tell anyone but I was even cutting out coupons and saving money at the grocery store. The coupon thing was a temporary moment of insanity, but I proved that I could do it. This was by far the most gratifying three weeks of my life. I wished like hell that I could quit work and take care of my kids forever.

It took a couple of weeks before the full impact of her death had sunk in. I had been so busy taking care of her and worrying about the kids that I really hadn't had a chance to think about what her loss would mean to me. I started listening to the tape of the memorial service numerous times each day and in the privacy of my back deck cried for her, for the kids and for myself. At this point I was praying that the old saying about time healing all wounds was true. During those three weeks I also spent some quality time with my yard. It was relaxing but each time, before I finished mowing the whole yard, I started feeling like I needed to hurry so that I could get one more load of laundry done and get supper started before the kids got home from school. Two years ago laundry was below scooping dog poop on my list of priorities, but now it is even higher than mowing. My transformation was maturing and I looked in the mirror and screamed, "I am not an animal!"

After Lisa died I started getting a lot of depressing things in the mail. The hospice was always sending me newsletters and articles that were designed to help me grieve. At the time I really wasn't in the mood for support groups and speeches, so I usually threw them away without reading them. It couldn't have been more than a month after the funeral when I started getting copies of a singles club newsletter. These people must read the obituaries every week, wait for a one month grace period to let the widow/ widower have a chance to get over their loss and then start inviting them to singles parties. At first the whole idea kind of ticked me off. I put these people in the same category as ambulance chasers and used car dealers. It made me so mad that I had to read it just to see what kind of things these outrageous people did. The more I read, the more ridiculous and funny it seemed. I had to laugh. The letter came with a list of all the members, complete with phone numbers. Judging by the names (i.e. Gertrude, Harold) I would have to guess that this was more of the geriatric crowd, which might explain the rush. Some of them might have been alone for a long time and needed some new blood to get them jump-started. Others just might not have much time to wait around. After reading the letters I threw them in the trash, but I couldn't stop thinking about how funny it was so I retrieved them from the trash, wiped off the coffee grounds and put them in my desk drawer.

One day, a Race for the Cure entry form showed up in my box. This was a harsh reminder of how quickly times change. Less than a year before Lisa had been in remission and felt good enough to run in this event. Now she was dead. There was no doubt that the kids and I were going to do this run. I was still deep in the middle of my Superhero, ("I can do everything, kick ass and take names") attitude.

Unlike the prior race (when I was in such dismal physical condition that I about died on the course), this year I was going to try to cross the finish line running instead of crawling. The kids were excited as well. They immediately started giving me the play-by-play of last year's race. They remembered the food, the big pink water bottles, and the door prizes they won after the race. They also all remembered how they ran out to meet their Mom and finished the run with her. That was a special moment for us all and they smiled and jumped up and down as they all at the same time gave me their version of how it happened.

Like the year before, the kids were so excited that they bounced out of bed on the day of the race and quickly got dressed. We followed Lisa's parents to the race site, as they were going to do the run again this year as well. It was a cool morning, perfect for running. When we got there it was very similar to the big party at the prior year's race. Tents with food and drinks were set up, music was booming over the loudspeakers and some aerobics instructors were leading a large group of people in some pre-race warm-ups. The kids immediately ran to the tent with the donuts and I went to find the registration forms.

When I found the registration tent I saw the two separate stacks of pink paper that were to be pinned to the backs of our shirts. The piece of paper we wore the last race read "In Support of." The paper we were going to wear this race read "In Memory of." Seeing this made my stomach hurt and I was worried how the kids would react. I waved them over from stuffing their faces with little donuts so I could get their signs pinned on. They each wanted to write "Mom" on their own and genuinely felt proud to be a part of this event in honor of their mother. Their ability to enjoy the moment picked me up off the pavement and my stomachache disappeared. At least until the race started.

The difference between this race and the last one was how differently people reacted to the kids when they saw the "In Memory of Mom" on their backs. Instead of talking to the kids, people would just look at them with that "Oh, you poor child," look. Then they would glance briefly up at me and walk away. The last thing I wanted was a bunch of pity for the kids or me. I don't think the kids noticed, as they were too wrapped up in seeing what they could eat or drink next.

The men's race started, and I was determined to stay

relaxed and not hyperventilate like I did the year before. That proved impossible. The horn blast started the runners in motion and soon I found myself running out of control with the leaders. My emotions had managed to overcome my efforts and my lungs started to burn and my stomach got a large cramp in it. I slowed down and even thought about walking. But every time I wanted to quit I thought about all the pain Lisa had endured and what a baby I was for even thinking about quitting. Somehow I ran through the pain, and before long I felt as though I had a new body. My mind cleared up, my lungs started breathing easily and my legs felt strong. I felt as though I had to pass every runner wearing an "In Support of" sign. I wanted them to see my "In Memory of " sign and I wanted to kick their butts because I thought I had more of a right to be there than they did. You might say that I was a bitter man. Why couldn't I have the same attitude as my kids? When I was finally able to see the finish line I was really cruising and I didn't want it to end. I sprinted the last 50 yards passing as many "In Support of" runners as I could.

The kids had a great time doing the one-mile fun run. They felt very cool with their race numbers pinned to the front of their official "Race for the Cure" T-shirts they received as runners. These kids just kept on seeing the simple, bright side of things. Without trying they forced me to recognize the positive feelings and support that permeated the event. But I was still a bit too raw to participate fully in the day's activities. The kids begged me to stay for the raffle like we had the previous year, but I was in no mood to hang around any longer than I had to. This was only about six weeks after Lisa died and it was more of an emotional strain than we could have imagined. Lisa's parents and I just wanted to go home. So we did.

In the months to follow my biggest fear was Christmas. I was afraid that no matter how hard I tried, Christmas was going to be a depressing, sad and mad experience for me and for the kids.

No matter how much I planned, I had never succeeded in avoiding that last minute Christmas shopping panic. To make matters worse, because of my ego and my need to prove to myself and to everyone else in the world that I could do this alone, I refused to accept any help. People had been helping so much and for so long that I wanted it to stop.

The kids and I picked out a tree and brought it home for the traditional decorating and hanging of the stockings as we always had done in the past with their mom. "Hey Dad, what are we going to do with Mom's stocking this year?" Samantha asked as she pulled it out of the box. It caught me completely off guard and my first reaction was to have her put it back in the box but I could tell that this might not be the best approach. When in doubt, ask the kids; it had gotten me this far.

"What do you guys think? Should we put mom's stocking out by the fireplace for Christmas?"

"Yeah, put it out," they all screamed.

"Then we can split the candy that Santa leaves for her," said the sweet-toothed Emily. The kids all cheered at that suggestion and once again they turned a potential disaster into a positive experience. We finished decorating the tree laughing and singing Christmas songs.

When Christmas Eve arrived I was still buying gifts and hadn't wrapped a single present. All the gifts under the tree were from relatives, and Santa still needed to work his magic. It was going to take a Christmas miracle. We went to the candlelight service at church, which meant that by the time we got home it was already very late. I got the kids to bed at about 11 o'clock and went to work wrapping presents. First I ran out of scotch tape and had to use duct tape. Then I ran out of wrapping paper and resorted to wrapping with cut up grocery sacks. At about 4 a.m. I finally finished and went to bed. I was just about asleep when I realized that the kids had put out celery (we were out of carrots, of course), cookies and milk for Santa and the damn reindeer. I needed to leave a note thanking them for the goodies. The note I wrote went just like this:

Dear Donners:

I met the most beautiful and nicest angel last night when I stopped at your house. She said that she was your mom and that she watched over you all the time. She also told me about your plan to leave her Christmas stocking out and trick me into filling it with candy so that you guys can split it. She thought that was funny and told me to go ahead and put some goodies in her stocking because you are such great kids and she loves you very much.

p.s. Thanks for the milk and cookies, but the reindeer would rather have carrots next time, not celery.

Santa

Even though Samantha knew there was not really a Santa Claus, she liked the note so much that she took it to school and read it at show and tell. That note is still pinned to her bulletin board today.

Wiped out as I was, the kids unanimously agreed and literally said that this was the greatest Christmas ever. That made me sad for Lisa's sake, but made me very proud of myself for being able to pull this off and make it a good memory instead of a bad one. As I think back on how my minor childhood traumas seemed to have impacted my personality and my behavior, I wonder how these truly traumatic experiences will affect these kids. My hope is that unlike my experiences (where my memory of the end result was how I was laughed at and ridiculed), their memories will be more positive. Emily won't think about how sad she was when her balloon popped but rather about how her siblings rallied around her and shared their balloons. Samantha hopefully will forget about how upset her mom was when she realized she was missing her birthday, and remember how happy her mom was to watch her open that present. She should also feel good about how her friends accepted her mom and didn't act like she was a freak even though she was bald, in a wheelchair and had a long tube running from her nose all the way into the bedroom. I hope Ben forgets about the disappointment of missing his mom's spirit and remembers the big hug I gave him and the reassurance that she was already an angel. Gaven, she was so young, who knows what she will remember. She was Lisa's baby and the only one that Lisa didn't mind rubbing her hairless head. Time will tell, but I hope the positive things are what they take away most from these unfortunate experiences.

From the very beginning of this horrible adventure, Lisa and I were determined to do everything we could to save the children. To make sure that their lives were not going to be ruined. Never during this whole ride did I think that the kids were going to be the ones saving me. They did so time and time again.

A Wrestling Match With the Devil

There I was, standing on this rocky mountain top, in the middle of a dense fog. My hair was shoulder length and black like the mane on a horse. Tied loosely around my neck was a long black cape, which hung down to the tops of my black, leather boots. Before you get the wrong idea, I was not wearing a thong with matching whip. I was wearing pants and a shirt which were gray and not worth mentioning. Anyway, in this dream, the wind was blowing hard and my face was pointed directly into it. My hair and cloak were flapping behind me as the gale gradually intensified. It was a powerful force and I couldn't tell if I was trying to stand up against it or absorb it. Either way it felt good, and I was trying to see how much my body could take. Then, without warning, a tremendous blast of wind came barreling into me, hitting me square in the chest, and knocking me flat on my back. Slowly I picked myself up, shook my head, and it was over. This had come to me in my sleep many times, beginning about the time that Lisa's morphine-induced hallucinations began. It recurred sporadically for months even after she died.

When I think back on Lisa's death and the trail of events leading up to it, there is no doubt that the two months prior to her dying were by far the most grueling and exhausting experience my mind and body had ever been through. When she was at home, unable to walk or go to the bathroom without help, needing oxygen round the clock and whacked out on drugs, it got so hard that I truly was afraid for my own physical and mental health. I was pushed way beyond any limitations that I could have imagined. During those two months I averaged somewhere between three and four hours of sleep, which might have been enough if they were quality, uninterrupted hours. But that was not the case. The major problem was that Lisa was like a baby who had her days and nights mixed up. While I was at work, Lisa's parents, her sister and various other family members would be at my house taking care of her and the kids. While I was gone, Lisa slept most of the morning and a good part of the afternoon. It seemed that shortly after I got home from work she would slowly start to come to life. We would get her up and feed her some supper and she would spend some time with the kids. This activity tired her out and she would sleep for a bit, maybe from eight o'clock to ten or eleven. During this time I would get the kids bathed and put to bed, and everyone else who had put in a very long day would go home for some well-deserved rest.

Every night I would slip into my bed and pray that she

would stay asleep. It never happened. First she would sit up, swing her dysfunctional legs over the edge of the bed (forgetting that she couldn't walk and that she was hooked up to all kinds of tubes) and try to go to the bathroom. Ding, ding, ding and the ring announcer would bellow out over the loud speaker that was duct taped to my head, "Let's get ready to rummm-bbbble!"

I learned to sleep lightly or not at all. When she sat up on the edge of her bed I had to move fast and grab her before she tried to stand, because she would surely fall. One such time, when she was still almost able to walk short distances using her walker, I found her lying half-naked on the bathroom floor, sobbing as she had wanted so badly to be able to use a regular toilet, instead of the port-a-potty, and more importantly to do it herself. She felt so helpless. Later that night, during a moment of sanity she said, "If I asked you to, would you kill me?" This question, as horrible as it seems, did not come as a big surprise to me.

"If I could do it without the risk of going to jail and leaving the kids without a mom or a dad, I might be able to do it," I said gravely. Bottom line is that at times we treat dogs with more respect than we do people. (Dr. K, do you have a web site?) Where is the dignity, especially for someone like Lisa, in dying this way? This cow has a way of stripping you of everything, especially your dignity, and it was no wonder that one of her biggest fears was being remembered as a sickly, helpless, and hairless crazy woman.

The bathroom attempts would go on throughout the night. Most of the time I would get her on the potty only to have her sit, unable to go. After two or three of these false alarms she would seem to relax, and I would lay back down and hope to get some sleep.

There I was, standing alone on a rock in the dense fog, my chin pointed directly into a wind which was tugging hard on my thick hair and cape, as it tried to pull me to the ground. But I endured what seemed to be the worst of it until this massive force came shooting almost straight down, hitting my shoulders and driving them to the rock directly beneath my boots. There was a scream coming from far off of someone in agony, so I jumped up to help. The fog lifted and there was Lisa, sitting up in bed, frantically yelling at me to make the pain stop while pushing the magic morphine button. It took a few long minutes for the drugs to take control again and I was forced to hold onto her until the pain passed to keep her from ripping her tubes out of the port-a-catheter in her chest. Even in her weakened state she was very strong. It was like wrestling with the devil, but I held tight until the pain demons relaxed and rested.

One night I woke to see blood squirting out of her drug line that had somehow become unattached. Lisa had rolled over on the tube and pulled it loose. I found the loose end underneath her body and reattached it to the end with the blood shooting out. There was a big red sticker on the phone with the hospice hot line number on it, which I quickly dialed to have them send out a nurse. It was about 3 a.m. when the on-call nurse arrived. He quickly changed out all her tubing, and restored everything to normal. I didn't want him to leave. It was so nice to have someone sane to talk with even at that late hour. Of course, Lisa slept the whole time he was there.

Somehow I had managed to harden myself to these scenes, or maybe it wasn't hardening as much as it was just pure fatigue. Once again I tried to get some sleep knowing that there was a good chance that the extra dose of morphine would start playing funny tricks on her mind and we would be at it again.

"Emily, quit bouncing that ball. You have to give it back to whomever it belongs to. Ben, get off of that before you fall and get hurt, and Samantha, you can't wear those shoes with that dress. Now go and change." It's 3:30 in the morning and I'm shocked out of my almost sleep with Lisa calling out to the kids that she thinks are running around in our room. Her motherly instincts run deep; even in her hallucinations she was on their butts. Then she pointed over to the chair in the corner of our room and started yelling, "Stop that. You two stop doing that, it's so stupid."

"Who are you yelling at?"

"It's Andre Agassi and Brooke Shields. Don't you see them David?"

She called me David more than my own name. David is

one of her brothers who was a nurse in the Air Force. She used to talk to him whenever she needed medical advice or verbal ammunition to fire at unsuspecting nurses. Anyway, I answered her, "No I can't see them, but I wish I could. I would tell them to go home so I could get some sleep."

On more than one occasion she would swear that there was someone looking in our bedroom window and make me go check. I'm not easily spooked, but in the middle of the night looking out my window to verify that no one was standing out there, especially at the request of a hallucinating partner, was a bit scary. Who knows what she was seeing? Could it be the Grim Reaper checking in to see if she had given up yet? If it was, he probably thought, "Damn, doesn't she know when to quit?"

It seemed that with the first hint of dawn she would settle down and konk out and so would I. At 6:15 a.m. my alarm would go off and I would drag myself to the shower, and get dressed for work just in time to see Lisa's dad cutting through the back yard toward my deck signifying the end of my shift. About 30 minutes later her mom would pull in the driveway just in time for me to head to work. This routine lasted for about eight weeks. I didn't know it at the time but my sleep habits would never be the same.

Work was the place I went to escape the physical reality. If I was lucky I would, if even for a brief moment, find something interesting enough to allow me to escape the mental reality. My rubber ball of a career was rolling around on the floor, but at least it was moving. My bosses allowed me to hang around so I could draw a paycheck and keep my insurance. If anyone else had been doing nothing like I was, they would have been canned. I knew that and was grateful. These were good people.

Aside from the obvious financial benefits, work had provided a couple of other elements that were critical to my survival. First, there was my friend Bruce who listened to my ramblings as I relived the previous night's wrestling matches. It was important for me to have someone to tell this to other than Lisa's parents. They worried enough about me as it was. Bruce was a good listener and gave me the sympathetic pep talks that I needed to keep moving. He kept suggesting that I take advantage of the company's good insurance plan and have the hospice provide a nighttime nurse to take care of Lisa so that I could get some sleep. I knew that this was good advice, but I could not let anyone else take care of her. I was afraid I would miss something really important and then forever regret not being there. There also was a big part of me that, for some reason, needed to do this by myself. Something was pulling me to this unbearable challenge as a form of soul-searching. It reminds me of my dream where this force keeps knocking me flat on my ass but I keep getting back up. Maybe it's just some dumb macho thing that would lead an 'ist' person to nod his head in recognition.

The quiet time at work allowed me to realize that I was a health risk, a walking time bomb, or a prime candidate for spontaneous human combustion. Yes, I was about to explode. I could literally feel the pressure throbbing inside my head, and when I told this to Bruce he walked me down to one of those do-it-yourself blood pressure machines. Just putting my arm in the inflatable cuff made my heart race. The read out on the machine indicated that I was approaching the danger zone.

Bruce looked at me and told me that I needed to do something different or I was going to beat Lisa to the grave. It was all too obvious what had happened. The cow had lifted its tail once again and deposited a dump-truck sized load of stress on me. There was, of course, the stress of Lisa's illness and the reality that I would be left with four kids to care for. Over the past few months my diet had gone to hell, I had stopped exercising, I was getting almost no sleep, I had people in my house all the time, and most alarmingly I had stopped drinking beer.

I could do nothing about many of the things causing my health deterioration. But the things that I could control I decided to fix. I started taking short runs in the evening and sneaking off to the gym during work at least two times a week. All those nutritious things I was buying out of the vending machines were taken off the menu. Finally (and I truly believe this was the most important change I made), I started having my nightly beer again. Lisa's parents don't drink and I felt a bit self-conscious popping open a beer when they were around. When they started to be around all the time, I quit drinking altogether. Having a beer was my way of washing down the day's crud, and it gave me a moment of carefree relaxation. I didn't realize how therapeutic it had been for me until I quit. So under the guise of good health I started drinking again. When the kids were in bed, Lisa's parents had gone home, and Lisa was sleeping, I could go out on my back deck, look up at those beautiful Kansas stars and pour a cold beer into my weary body. It slid down my throat and I could feel it as it made its way down to my toes and fingertips. My eyes would close instinctively as I took a deep breath and forgot where I was for one or two minutes. Slowly my eyes would open, as my mind savored the last moment of its vacation. Then I would chug the rest of the beer and head back in through those doors. Maybe I should make a beer commercial.

One of those nights, not long after Lisa had died, I was out on the deck in the company of my beer when I opened my eyes to see Samantha running frantically around inside the house. Quickly, I went inside and grabbed her. She was very frightened, "Daddy, I came downstairs and couldn't find you. I thought you had left." I suppose I had, in a sense. My beer break let me go just far enough to ensure that I wouldn't lose it completely. Samantha's fear was not surprising. In fact it made perfect sense. The question "What happens to us if you die, Daddy?" was a good one, and I'm sure it was somewhere in her mind as she ran through the house.

One of the stress inducers affecting my health was the constant stream of people flowing through my house. This may not seem like a terribly stressful situation. In fact, given the circumstances, one could argue that the extra help would relieve stress. Sounds reasonable, but there is a difference between wanted help and needed help. I grew up in an environment that taught me to go to school, get a decent job and take care of my family. If there was any way that I could take care of my problems without asking for help, I found it. Even if it was more costly, took more time or was totally inconvenient, I wanted to do it myself. Right or wrong, in my simple, demented mind it was a sign of failure to ask for help. Consequently, it was driving me crazy to have help constantly milling around. What really bothered me (and created the stress) was that I could do nothing about it. In my perfect fat, dumb and happy life I would never need help from anyone; it simply wouldn't be necessary. Of course, I know now that everyone needs a little help now and then, and I'll accept it gratefully as long as I feel that I will have the opportunity to pay the helper back at some point. It's just not natural, however, to need help almost continuously for two or three years. Not that anyone ever expected anything in return (because they didn't) but I had a hard time figuring how I was ever going to repay any of this.

After a while, coming home from work and always see-ing someone else's car in my driveway made me angry. There was no one to be angry at, but every now and then I would take it out on the very people who were there helping. These people were my family and friends who were there on their own equally valuable time to help me and my family, and getting mad at them was just plain wrong. But I couldn't help it.

As I was struggling with my situation, I learned a couple of valuable lessons. These lessons did not come easily, but we all were in uncharted waters. When various family and friends came to help, I had certain expectations as to what kind of help was needed and I figured everyone should know my expectations with-out my having to communicate them. Of course when things weren't done 'right' I got angry and I'm sure I acted like a pouty baby sometimes. The other grotesque error I made was that I not only expected people to know what was needed, I expected them to be capable of doing it regardless of their skills. My dad was a classic victim in this regard. For a long time I was angry with him because when he and Mom would come to visit with the notion of helping, he was totally lost. The basic kind of help that was needed revolved around taking care of kids and daily household chores such as laundry, cooking, cleaning, or giving baths. This was stuff that he had never done because my mom always did it. Not that he was one of those lazy couch potato guys. He wasn't. When I was growing up he was working 70 hours a week and understandably did not have time to help with these daily household duties. If the washing machine needed fixing or the lawn needed mowing he would jump and do it. He was a project guy, and I just didn't have the time to think of any projects for him. Certainly not ones that would keep him busy for the two weeks that they would stay.

On one occasion he was standing around watching a 24-hour news channel on the boob tube while I was scurrying around sweeping, mopping, picking up toys, and emptying the dishwasher. It was all I could do not to explode, but instead I just picked up the toys and threw them into the toy box and stormed out of the room. A couple of days later he decided to go home and leave Mom to fly home by herself later. He made up some excuse about a doctor's appointment but also added that he felt like he wasn't being much help. I was sorry and sad that he felt that way, as it really wasn't his fault. But at the time it was more stressful than helpful to have him around and he understood that.

My mistake was wanting him to be a different person and to do things that were not in his nature. We all have our strengths and weaknesses and we either have it in us to be a certain way or we don't. It was wrong of me to expect people to walk into this pressure-filled situation and feel comfortable doing things that they weren't good at. I was making them jump out of the frying pan and into a very hot fire. My dad would have walked to the moon and back if I had asked him to. Just knowing that should have been enough for me, but at the time there was no way I could see the forest for the trees, or the herd for this cow.

When I got ticked off at my family for failing to know what I wanted them to be doing, I would put on my moppin' socks and proceed to sweep and mop the kitchen floor. The cleanliness of the floor was in direct proportion to my level of anger. I believe the cleanest my floor ever got was the day before the funeral. I had just finished bathing all four kids and putting them to bed when I came downstairs where some of my family were sitting in the family room watching television. For some reason the sight of them all relaxing while I was still working made me kind of mad. So I went into the laundry room to fold some clothes and start another load. As I was walking through the kitchen with an armload of clothes I noticed that the floor was still dirty from dinner. There they sat, munching on ice cream and watching some stupid show. They really didn't even notice me walking heavily back and forth on my way to and from the kitchen. I was getting pissed, so I went and got my moppin' socks on and grabbed a broom. After I finished sweeping the floor for the third time, they were all still sitting there watching The Three Stooges and laughing hysterically. "Hey Mooselips, why don't you come and watch the Stooges with us," yelled one of my brothers.

Frothing at the mouth, I grunted back, "I would love to but

the floor is still a mess from dinner," as I quickly started mopping with intent to kill. Luckily for all, they decided it was time to go to bed just before I mopped a hole in the linoleum. They said good night and I made a sour face and nodded. Was I being a brat who wanted some big-time suck up sympathy, or what? Maybe I was justified in being upset but it wasn't serving any purpose. Probably the best thing I could have done for myself and everyone around me would have been to sit down and watch the Stooges. The floor would have appreciated the reprieve as well.

Lisa's family was quite different. They were more like the guards at Buckingham Palace. With tightly pursed lips, they would constantly review Lisa's drug schedule or review the calendar for the upcoming appointments or kids activities. To be quite honest they made me a bit nervous. I was afraid that I was going to screw something up or forget something important. This of course was not their intent; it was more a sign of my weariness and my waning self-confidence. There were times when I truly did not know what I was doing. They often knew better what Lisa wanted or needed, and I found myself second-guessing many things that should have been no-brainers. They were always there, and they definitely didn't need anyone to tell them what to do, they just did whatever was necessary. Lisa was their daughter, after all. Sometimes I wondered if there was a pecking order in cases like this. Did I, as the husband, have the right to tell them it was time for them to go home each night, or could they justifiably say that it was their daughter and stay as long as they wanted? This was never an issue, as they seemed to understand and respect what I wanted and why. They frequently asked if I needed a break at night, as they knew that I was wrestling with Lisa and not getting much sleep. There were times when I was tempted to let them spend the night in my place, but I just had to do it myself.

The week before she died, things got to be unbearable. I was getting even less sleep, three hours at the most, and I was wondering how much longer she was going to hang on like this and how much longer I could hang on. Finally I conceded, and agreed to call the hospice and ask for a nurse to spend one night so that I could get some sleep. What I really needed and prayed for was some kind of divine intervention to put a stop to this one way or the other.

I was somewhat anxious before the hospice nurse arrived, as I really didn't know what to expect. What kind of person would do this sort of thing for a living? Would she be able to handle the wild ride that Lisa was going to put her through? This I had to see. Surely she was going to need my help at some point.

The doorbell rang and there she stood. I looked but I did not see a car. As I opened the door she greeted me with a small but comforting smile and stepped inside without being asked; she knew she was welcome here. She shook my hand with a firm hand that was soft and somehow both warm and cool at the same time, almost as if they could be whatever was needed. She mentioned her name casually as if it didn't matter, and I sensed that after this night I would never see her again. Her hair was brown and cut short to about an inch in length, possibly to make the hairless cancer patients more comfortable. From the moment I saw her I tried to guess how old she was, but she had the look of someone who was in a holding pattern. Later I would let my curiosity get the best of me and break the rule of never asking a woman her age and ask her point blank, "How old are you?"

"Old enough to be a grandmother," she said without batting an eye.

Without asking she glided past me towards the bedroom. If I had not seen her feet moving I would not have been able to tell she was walking, as her upper body barely flinched. I followed her to Lisa's bed where she immediately sat down on its edge and started stroking Lisa's hands and head and telling her how beautiful she was. She asked me a few basic questions about our kids and then went back to holding Lisa's sleeping hand and talking softly to her. I asked her if she needed anything and she said no.

This was supposed to be the night for me to get some sleep, but I couldn't. I made some coffee and sat down at the kitchen table to write in my journal and read. Later I walked back to the bedroom to check on Lisa and ask the nurse if she wanted

147

any coffee. The nurse was sitting in the rocking chair, as still as can be, with her hands clasped on her lap while she gazed at a peaceful Lisa. The room was dimly lit by a night light in the bathroom and a small reading lamp next to the rocker. The light by the chair appeared to be trapped inside a transparent egg around her. I stood there mesmerized until she spoke, "Yes, some coffee would be nice."

At midnight I felt compelled to bake some chocolate chip cookies. Don't get too impressed; they were the pre-made dough kind that came in the shape of a log that you glob off with a spoon onto a cookie sheet and throw in the oven. They may not taste as good as homemade but the smell is good enough for me. I brought her more coffee and some hot cookies. Lisa stirred a bit, probably from the smell of the chocolate, and she yelled out a couple of times. The nurse went to her side and quickly soothed her with a comforting voice and warm hands. Then the nurse looked right at me as I stood helplessly in the doorway and said, "She's going to be all right." The way she said that made it sound like she knew something that I did not know. She sounded so sure of herself that I suddenly felt relieved and relaxed enough to go and lay down on the couch. It was 4 a.m.

Just before 6 a.m. I woke up feeling very rejuvenated, even though I had only been asleep for a couple of hours. The nurse was putting on her sweater and getting ready to leave. Her shift was scheduled from 6 p.m. to 6 a.m. I felt kind of silly because Lisa slept the whole night, but all she said was how beautiful Lisa was and thanked me for the coffee and cookies. In the blink of an eye she was gone. She didn't have a car, and I think someone picked her up at the corner. After she left, I went back to my room and sat down in the chair she had been sitting in and got this weird sense that something miraculous had happened there. Maybe she was like a horse whisperer for people or maybe something more, I don't know, but her presence had affected us.

Lisa's mom and dad arrived right on schedule and I headed off to work. For some unknown reason I felt an urgent need to train this woman in my office on the one thing that I had been doing, as if I wasn't going to be around for awhile. After a few last minute instructions I hurried home for lunch and to give Lisa some additional medication which supplemented the morphine. When I arrived, our regular hospice nurse was there and she told me that there had been a significant change in Lisa's health. Her heart rate and breathing rate had started to drop. I had read in the fun facts brochure about death that this development generally signaled the beginning of the end. It was as if Lisa had finally decided it was okay to let it go. She had the same look on her face as when the night nurse had been talking to her and rubbing her skin. I don't know what the nurse said to her but it sure seemed to have worked.

During my short early morning nap, I had a dream. In my

dream I was lying in my bed and Lisa was in hers. Hovering over me were six angelic figures. Then five of them drifted over to Lisa's bed while one remained for just a moment over me before finally joining the others. That night, when Lisa's dad called me down from my 'your mom might die tonight' talk with the kids, I rushed into my bedroom to find six people all standing around Lisa's bed. Moments later she was gone.

A Broken Promise

It was a perfect sweatshirt and blue jeans fall evening. The kids and I were on the back deck playing with Dusty our golden retriever. Lisa had given me Dusty a few months after Samantha was born, probably so I could have a baby to take care of too. We all took a moment to admire another one of those incredible Kansas sunsets. In Kansas, because it is so flat and nothing obstructs your view except the high voltage wires, the sunsets seem to last forever. This sunset was more spectacular than usual as it lit up the feathery wisps of clouds with pinks, reds, oranges and lavenders. Gaven, who was sitting on my lap, pointed to the horizon and said, "Mom really did a good one didn't she Dad?" After their mom died and surely went to heaven to be an angel, the kids were curious as to what she would do up there. I told them that when she wasn't busy watching them she probably had a regular job, kind of like we do down here, except it would be something fun. Samantha had once remarked on how pretty a particular sunset was and thought that maybe her mom had some part in making sunsets. The other kids were happy to latch onto this notion, and from that point on that was their mom's job: Queen of Sunsets.

Lisa had been gone for a couple of months and things were going remarkably well for the kids. They were doing great in school, singing in the church choir, making friends and seeing their grandparents every day.

As for me, considering the circumstances, things were also going pretty well. The city was familiar to me, as I had lived and worked there right after college. This was also where Lisa and I met, so there were a lot of good memories floating around, and some of our old friends still lived there. Work was tolerable, and actually a good place to go and get away from the house. My morning schedule was a bit tight, getting the older girls to a before-school care program and then dropping the little guys off at their preschool halfway across town. If I hit the traffic lights just right I could get to work almost on time. Then at the end of the workday I had to sneak out a bit early and really hustle to pick up everyone. Taking care of my kids was what I wanted to do more than anything. No one at work ever questioned my leaving, and if they had I wouldn't have cared.

Lisa's parents were happy to be able to see their grandchildren almost daily and were always willing to help out whenever I needed anything. It was very comforting knowing that family was only a sidewalk away. There were other relatives in town as well.

Lisa's aunt and uncle lived a few miles away, and as sure as Thursday came every week so did they with a huge meal. Typically it was grown-up food that my kids hadn't yet developed a taste for, and it came in portions big enough to feed the whole neighborhood. It took at least an hour just to empty the remains into many containers so I could clean the huge pots and pans it came in. They were such sweet and generous people that I could never tell them to stop or that a bag of cheeseburgers and French fries would be the perfect meal for us. The kids' aunt, Lisa's sister, lived a few hours away and would pop into town on weekends every once in a while. The kids enjoyed being with this person who looked and sounded a lot like their mom.

A few of Lisa's longtime childhood friends lived in town as well, and occasionally would drop by or offer to take the kids for an afternoon so that I could do something by myself. It was such a luxury to go to the grocery store without the four Tasmanian Devils knocking people and carts into the next aisle. It was a relief to hear the voice over the loud speaker say, "Cleanup in aisle four," and not have to check what aisle I was in.

We were living in a really nice neighborhood, and the house was roomy, with a large finished basement, which functioned as a playroom for the kids. The backyard connected to the community playground and there was a huge, wide-open field where many of the neighborhood kids came to play.

The sun was shining, the sky was blue, the birds were chirping and all things considered nothing was going wrong. Why then did I feel like shit?

I'm sure that all you junior 'ist' people are saying, "Well, you just lost your wife and you are supposed to feel like shit." That is so obvious that I was able to tell the difference between my grieving and other things that were screwed up. It's these other things that were making me feel like shit.

Everything that was going good had a flip side that was not quite so good. The kids hated the fact that they had to go to before-school care. If their mom were alive they wouldn't have to. As much as they hated it, I hated it twice as much for them. It was also such a panic every morning to get all four kids fed, dressed and loaded into the car early enough so that I could get to work on time. They were all still very young and required quite a lot of assistance. To make matters worse, I made whatever each of them wanted for breakfast each morning. It was the least I could do, and if I ever lost my job I knew I could work anywhere as a short order cook.

Lisa's parents had offered to help out by driving or coming over in the mornings and getting the kids on the bus. They actually did this for a short bit, but I could see the sadness on their faces as they walked into this house. This house, where they had spent so much time watching their daughter die. It just wasn't fair.

The house, Lisa's dream house, had for me become more

of a nightmare house. It was not possible for me to walk into my bedroom without having flashbacks of her and the torture she went through. It's amazing that I was able to sleep in there at all. Sometimes it was definitely creepy. After she died I left all her stuff just as it was, clothes, shoes, chemo scarves, prosthesis, jewelry, everything. I just didn't want to deal with it. The kids seemed okay running around in the house, but it was hard to know what they were thinking. For them it seemed that being around their mom's stuff was comforting in a sad kind of way. Every once in a while Samantha would be in bed and just start crying. "What's wrong Samantha?" I would ask as I sat down on the edge of her bed.

"I don't know, I guess I just miss my mom."

"We all miss her, and its okay to cry anytime you want," I said as I wiped her nose with my sleeve.

Samantha missing her mother was extremely normal and would most likely have happened even if she hadn't been living among so many reminders of her mom, but it was a bit unsettling how everything in the house was exactly the same except that Mom was gone.

One morning I was sitting on my back deck enjoying my coffee, when a large piece of construction paper came floating down from Emily's bedroom window. The note was neatly written and fully illustrated, it read, "I hat you Dad." I shouted up at her window, "Don't you mean I hate you Dad?"

Just then mother Samantha came scurrying from around front. "Dad, Emily is running down the street," she yelled in a panic. My sweet Emily was running away from home. I jumped on my bike and caught up to her about a block from the house and pedaled up along side. "Where ya going Emily," I asked in a non-interested tone. She looked at me with sadly determined eyes and increased her pace. She looked over again and noticed how easily I was able to stay up with her and realized the futility of her flight. She smiled sheepishly and stopped. I got off my bike and we walked home together. It was obvious that she was angry, but she, unlike Samantha, couldn't (or wouldn't) talk about it. Her mode of communication was through her drawings, which always included portions of our house as a setting. She was very young and this behavior was probably considered normal, but I wondered if the house was throwing fuel on the fire. They really had nowhere to go that the death of their mom wasn't staring them in the face. School, church, friends and relatives were all constant reminders. Where could they go to escape for needed breaks from reality? Or was it better that they were forced to confront it and deal with it every day? An 'ist' I am not, so I crawled around on my hands and knees feeling my way through the dark maze of uncertainty.

In retrospect, I made a mistake by trying to protect the kids from situations that might make them angry or sad. Maybe it wasn't that I was protecting them as much as I was steering them away from these emotions because they made me feel uncomfortable. One of my stronger personality traits is my ability to internalize these emotions and hold them in until they (hopefully) go away. Rarely do I ever openly express my anger or sadness, and therefore it is not natural for me to encourage these expressions as acceptable forms of behavior. How is that for some 'ist' lingo?

Ben had a different way of looking at things. Being only four years old might have had something to do with that. One day he was lying on his back stretched out across the top of the stairs with his feet on the wall. As I stepped over him he blurted out of the blue, "We sure had Mom around for a pretty long time didn't we Dad?"

"Yes Ben, I suppose you're right. She was around for almost your entire life."

His comment surprised me. I realized that even though he was only four years old he didn't spend his whole day trying to see how long he could wait before peeing in his pants and trying to decide what kind of cereal he was going to have for breakfast. Probably for Gaven and Ben, because of how young they were, being around their mom's stuff all day and night was a positive thing, and seemed to help them keep the feeling of their mom alive.

For the most part my job was secure, the pay was decent and it provided good benefits, all of which I needed, but the work itself was totally boring and uninspiring to me. Especially after

Lisa's death I found it increasingly difficult to perform my job, as all the tasks seemed irrelevant in my newly reorganized list of priorities. Justifying putting my kids in special day care programs just so I could spend 8 hours a day looking at process flow diagrams on a computer screen and reading meaningless emails was damn near impossible to do. If Lisa and I hadn't cashed in her life insurance policy so we could afford to have kids then I might have been able to stay home and not work for a few years, or at least until they all were in school. If we hadn't started having kids we would have been able to afford the premiums on her policy, but then I wouldn't have needed it. I had been caught by Catch-22. The moral of this story is to buy as much life insurance as you can reasonably afford, and a little insurance would be better than no insurance, because it doesn't always happen to the other guy. Fat, dumb and happy people like myself have a tendency to get caught with our pants down.

The other thing making work impossible was that ever since Lisa's funeral my co-workers found me even more unapproachable than before. Was I always going to be known as the scary guy whose wife died, leaving him with their four motherless kids to raise on his own? My rubber ball career had rolled itself into a corner with no place to go.

My friends, who had also been Lisa's friends, treated me differently, or so it seemed. I made them feel rather uncomfortable, and sometimes when they saw me with the kids they would start to cry. It got to the point that no one asked me to do anything anymore, especially the couples we knew. Lisa's longtime childhood friends eventually stopped coming by or calling altogether.

The church we went to was warm and welcoming, but it was also the church where we were married and the church Lisa had attended her whole life. I couldn't go in there without having some elderly person come up to me and start telling me stories of how they remembered Lisa when she was little and how much my kids resembled her. Those comments were well-intended and appreciated, but it would have been nice to talk to about regular stuff with them every once in a while. It got so bad that I started dropping the kids off at Sunday school and sneaking off to a park or coffee shop to read or write in my journal.

It felt like I was living in a fishbowl. The kids and I were swimming around and around in one of those small goldfish tanks while the rest of the world was on the outside watching everything we did. "Oh look, he is going to the grocery store and all the kids are going with him and look what kind of food is in his cart. Does he cook? That poor man. Those poor kids." Every once in a while the thought of dating crossed my mind but it's hard to do from inside a fishbowl. Besides, whoever the lucky woman was would have to grow gills and be in the fishbowl with all of us. The Little Mermaid was already taken, so I decided to put my energy where it really belonged, on my kids.

I found myself developing a certain kind of inevitable paranoia whenever the kids and I were around Lisa's family. For example, if Ben were to haul off and slug Emily, I would say to myself, "Now what would Lisa do here?" I felt like they were watching to see if I was raising the kids the way Lisa would have wanted them to be raised. I tried to do this for a while, but I wasn't sure how she would do everything and it got confusing inside my little head. Once Lisa's sister came to stay at my house for the weekend so I could get away for a couple of days. When I got back she informed me that she whipped those kids into shape and they cleaned the whole house. "They should be helping you around the house more," she told me. She had them make a chores list for each day of the week. That was something that Lisa might have done, but I obviously wasn't doing it. There was no doubt in my mind that this would be a good thing for them to be doing and I appreciated her effort, but because of how thin I was stretched I had to pick which battles I wanted to fight, and this was not one of them. For the time being it was more time efficient and less stressful for me to make their beds than to fight with them about doing it. Unfortunately, it was difficult for people to appreciate my situation completely if they weren't living it eight days a week.

Wherever we showed up, the stress level in the room jumped. We were walking, breathing reminders of some bad stuff.

160

No one blamed us for anything, but it seemed that we had an almost unavoidable way of bringing people outside of their comfort zone.

The first big holiday after Lisa's death was Thanksgiving. I decided to avoid a potentially depressing situation by putting us all on an airplane and visiting my brother and his family in North Carolina. It was quite an adventure herding four little kids through an extremely busy O'Hare Airport, especially when all the girls had to go to the bathroom at the same time and the line, as usual for the women's restroom, was out the door. (You would think that someone would figure this out and quadruple the capacity of the women's facilities.) I ended up taking them all into the less crowded men's restroom and locked us all in one stall until everyone had gone potty. We were a very close family. The kids had never been on a plane before and were pretty much spellbound. We made it without incident. Of course it helps to have lots of gum and candy to throw at them the whole trip.

Thanksgiving was a big success. My brother has four kids as well and they are all about the same age as mine. The cousins all had a lot of fun being together and it felt more natural for me to be around my family.

I had been to North Carolina to visit my brother and his wife about a month prior to Thanksgiving, and while I was there we semi-seriously talked about how nice it would be if I moved there. This sounded kind of good to me, but there were two things that I thought were insurmountable hurdles. The first was finding a job that would pay enough for me to be able to afford living there. Not that I'm a derelict or anything, but I had worked for the same company my whole career and my skills were rather company-specific and not easily marketable.

The other hurdle was even bigger, and it had to do with a promise that I had made to Lisa before she died. She had gone through a ton of crap to get herself healthy enough to be able to move to Kansas for the sole purpose of having her parents around to help take care of her kids in case the cow came back to visit. She told me that one of her fears was that after she died I would pack up and move someplace. She knew me pretty well, but I told her that I would never do that. I promised her that I would stay put. It wasn't this dramatic movie scene where she was on her deathbed making me swear on her grave that I would keep this promise, but it was something that was really important to her and I did not take it lightly. When the topic of moving came up, I had to remind everyone that I had made this pledge to Lisa and that I wouldn't feel right breaking my promise.

As we all know, where there is a will there is a way…a way to rationalize almost anything if you want something bad enough. Our rationalization discussion led us to think that what Lisa worried about was that I would move someplace and not have the family support that we needed. But if I were to move to a town that had good family support, like where my brother and his family lived, then it would be okay with Lisa. Convincing myself that Lisa would accept this would be easy compared to having to tell Lisa's parents that I would be moving and taking their daughter's children away from them.

I was conflicted about the whole idea, but I agreed to let my brother pass my resume´ around to people that he knew from work just to see what happened. Well, over the next month I got a couple of nibbles and when we came back for Thanksgiving I had arranged for a couple of informal interviews. I was starting to get scared and wondered if I was doing the right thing.

Nothing definite had come out of the interviews but I had my foot in the door. My rubber ball of a career rolled out of the corner hit a small pebble, got airborne and landed with a small bounce. My two biggest fears now were 1) that I would not get offered a job; and 2) that I would get offered a job. Nobody hires anyone between Thanksgiving and New Years, so I figured I had a little bit of time to figure out if moving was the right thing for me, the kids, and Lisa's parents.

When the kids and I were at my brother's for Thanksgiving I could feel that moving to North Carolina would be a very positive thing for all of us. I needed a change and some room to be myself again. Whoever that was. The kids had so much fun being around their cousins and they really latched onto their aunt. It was clear to me that they needed more of a daily influence from a female who was more their mom's age and energy level. Overall it felt very right. One of the many things I learned from my experience with the cow was that there are times when things just don't add up and nothing's clear. This is when you have to turn the noise in your brain way down low so that you can hear what your heart has to say. If your heart is good, there is a better than average chance that it will lead you down the right path.

What about Lisa's parents, how would they take this? The biggest issue would be that they knew Lisa wanted her kids to be close to them. Lisa knew that her parents would never let any harm come to her kids and that they had the time and resources to make sure of that. Most of all she knew that her parents loved her kids, and would sit on them like eggs until they hatched. The other issue was that these kids were what kept Lisa alive in some way for her parents. They could see her in the kids' eyes, in the way they moved and the way they smiled. Each of these kids could be a stubborn pain in the butt, which was also their daughter. Somehow, in my heart I knew that they would most likely understand my need to be happy and that through my happiness the kids would have a better chance at their own happiness.

I was not quite so sure of my heart to let it make this decision on its own, so I decided to get some other opinions. First, I talked to an 'ist' from hospice. They had been calling every month after Lisa died offering their services, and I kept declining because I didn't need to have an 'ist' tell me how to grieve. At the time I had this "I am a big boy and can do it myself" attitude. But now with this specific question in mind I surprised them during the next call by accepting their offer and scheduling an appointment.

The woman at the hospice was about my age and very pleasant. She was obviously book smart, but admitted to never having lived through an experience that even came close to mine. She was a good source for giving me the rule of thumb for moving to a new place after the death of a family member. Basically the rule was that you should not move for at least six months and never right before or during a holiday. This answer gave my brain what it wanted to hear. This exchange took up about the first 15 minutes of my scheduled one-hour appointment and for the next three hours I educated her on what I had learned over my summer vacation. It was actually very therapeutic to talk to an 'ist', who was a good listener.

The next person I talked with was Lisa's oldest brother who lived in California. He may have been Lisa's best friend, but she would just say that he was her brother who usually had very sound advice. He knew his parents as well as anyone and he was also very trustworthy. I knew that if I talked to him about the possibility of moving, he wouldn't spill the beans before I was ready. He thought that they would understand and support me in this move mainly because he knew that my brother and sister-in-law would be very supportive. His opinion carried a lot of weight, and I was relieved to have gotten a positive response. Two down, and one big one to go.

The final person I wanted to talk with was George, our pastor. He had been a friend of Lisa's family for a long time, and I had come to respect and value his opinion above just about all others. He came over to my house after the kids were in bed and (I thought) asleep. They must have felt his presence, because no sooner did we sit down and start talking than they each, one at a time, came to the balcony at the top of the stairs and said "Hi George." They loved George. He treated them like the special-people that they were and always said the right thing. "It's great to see you guys, but you need to help your dad out and go back to bed," he said, and they did it without a fuss. To them it was like having God tell them to go to bed.

"George, I really need to get out of this town. I'm having a hard time breathing here. I feel like there is something else that I am supposed to be doing and I need to go and find it."

"You are going through a lot of very big changes and this would be the perfect opportunity to follow your heart. You should trust your gut feelings."

"My gut feels like it is going to explode. The last thing I want to do is hurt anyone."

"I don't think anyone can question your dedication to your family and no one, especially Lisa's mom and dad, would think that you would do anything to put your kids at risk."

Right on, George.

The responses I had received from these sources gave me the confidence to pursue the move and new job opportunities. The problem was that once I got it in my head that I wanted to move, I became obsessed with the notion and could think of nothing else. My head and body were packed with so much nervous energy that I really couldn't work, I could barely sit in my chair and I spent a lot of time taking long walks around the factory. My bed time habits had been permanently altered and I was still only getting about four hours of sleep each night. I went to bed thinking about all that I would have to do to move, and as soon as I woke my mind picked up where it left off.

The only other person with whom I had discussed the move was my friend Bruce. He was impressed that I had the courage to pack up these four little kids and head off on an adventure, leaving the security of the company that I had been with for 15 years and the support of a really good family and church. He made it sound kind of scary and rightfully so, but I was on a mission and I had promised myself that I would never second-guess my decision. I felt a bit like the race car driver in the movie 'Gumball Rally' as he rips the rearview mirror off and throws it out the window saying

"What's behind me doesn't matter."

My biggest obstacle was finding a job. I needed to have an income. At first I had this idea that I was going to find the job to end all jobs. I was in no hurry. I really didn't have a time limit so I thought I could be picky and find the perfect job. Well, I found out that I'm not the patient person I thought I was. The more I thought about leaving, the sooner I had to leave. My philosophy changed to fit my building urgency. I decided that I simply needed to find an adequate job for transitional purposes, and then once I was living there I could look for a better one if necessary.

There was some interest coming from one of my Thanksgiving-time interviews. It was a job at a medical center for a major university and sounded very cool. Because of my recent experiences with hospitals and medicines the thought of working for a medical center was extremely appealing. The possibility of actually being able to directly help people got me rather excited. The lady I interviewed with asked for references and I gave her four, two of which were George and my old boss, Bill. They wrote letters of recommendations on my behalf and gave me copies of what they had written. Their letters were incredibly flattering and made me feel very good about myself. After reading these letters, even I would have hired me.

Now I had to play the waiting game, and even with my hard-won patience nothing could happen fast enough for me. The days turned into weeks, and I felt that if this job didn't pan out it surely would be the end of the world. My nights got shorter and shorter as I was so nervous and stressed that I could barely sleep. If I wasn't doing laundry or writing in my journal, I was on the phone or sending e-mails all over the country. My sister-in-law and Lisa's friend who also had breast cancer were a great help to me during this time of uncertainty. They were both very supportive and kept telling me that moving was the right thing for me to do.

Then one night something truly unexplainable and Twilight Zone-ish happened. It was somewhere between two and three o'clock in the morning and I was in the middle of a deep sleep. In fact it was one of those rare nights when I had actually been able to relax and had gone to bed before midnight. Maybe it had been that extra beer, but for whatever reason my brain took a break and decided it would be okay to chill out for a bit. Anyway, I awoke to the sound of voices coming from my family room. I was temporarily paralyzed, not moving a muscle and trying not to breathe so that I could hear who was out there. Then I heard music mixed in with the voices, like a marching band and I realized that the television was on. Whoever was out there was watching television. The hair on my neck (and there is quite a bit of it) was standing straight up as I crawled out of bed and walked to the family room. I turned on a light and found no one, only a blaring television set. Shaking a bit, I grabbed the remote, turned down the volume, and walked over to the set to see if I could figure out what had turned it on. There hadn't been an electrical storm, all the digital clocks in the house were set and weren't flashing, and I just couldn't figure it out. I even ran upstairs to check on the kids. They were all sleeping like rocks. No clues.

As I was about to shut the television off, I noticed what was on. It was the rerun of a basketball game that had been played the night before. What really blew my mind was that one of the teams playing was the university where I was trying desperately to get the job. This was too damn bizarre to be a coincidence. After a moment I composed myself, shook my head from side to side real fast like a dog after it first wakes up, turned off the game and went back to bed. It took me a little while to calm down but I finally fell back asleep. Then it happened again. I woke to the sound of the TV and it seemed even louder than the first time and the same basketball game was still on. Quickly I turned it back off and started looking around the room, up at the ceiling, out the window. I didn't see anything, but I sure did feel something funny. All I could think of was that she was there somewhere and that she knew.

Electric Angel

My eyes were watering, cheeks burning, nose dripping, lips numb, forehead frozen, teeth cracking and lungs in a state of shock. Yes, I was out for another one of those delightful winter runs in Kansas. The wind was whipping across every exposed part of my body, ripping through the multiple layers of clothing as if I was naked. Four o'clock in the morning is about the coldest time of day, and it was about 22 degrees with a wind chill that had to be somewhere below zero. Why would any sane person be running at 4 a.m. in sub-zero temperatures? (The key to this question is the word 'sane.') My answer, of course, is that this was one of the few times during the day that someone or something was not demanding or requiring my time. I probably wasn't a finalist for the father of the year award anyway, so leaving the kids unattended for those fifteen to twenty minutes probably wasn't going to cost me the prize. They are sound sleepers and never wake up at this time of day. Besides, my running course was a short loop that circled past my house every 3-4 minutes so I was never far away.

171

This run, though very short, was needed to clear my cluttered head, and give that nervous energy someplace to go. When I wake up anxious, as I had that morning, it is essential that I get outside for a bit of air. When the climate is rather extreme it makes me concentrate on breathing and not freezing to death, instead of things that I could do nothing about at that moment such as job interviews, selling my house, and organizing the kids' activities. On that particular morning, there were no clouds to insulate the earth, and because I had to bury my head down in my chest to keep the wind from shooting down my neck I hadn't noticed how bright the stars were shining. All I could think about was getting this over with so I could get back to the warmth of the gas heat and Mr. Coffee.

I was about halfway around on my third lap when a large jet flew overhead and I was compelled to look up and visualize myself wearing Bermuda shorts and doing the limbo down the aisle of the plane as it jetted me to the Bahamas. When I did this two shocking things happened. The first thing was that the wind came pouring down my neck like ice water out of a faucet. This should have prompted the quick return of my face to my chest, but out of the small, unfrozen corner of my eye I saw the second shocking thing. It was a large hole that opened up in the night sky. From that hole gushed a brilliant light resembling the burning tip of a sparkler on the Fourth of July. It was the Hale-Bopp comet. They had been talking about it on the news and in the paper, but I had never taken the time to see if I could find it. But there it was. Hale-Bopp had found me. The light was so pure and bright I would almost have believed that it was one of heaven's windows opening up to let the angels fly out for their nightly rounds on earth.

For a few moments I was frozen like a statue, not from the cold but from a paralysis caused by the light of the comet. It made me warm all over and as I broke free from its spell and started to run again I twisted my neck around a few degrees short of 180 and even ran sideways to keep Hale-Bopp in my sight for as long as possible. The skies in the East were starting to lighten, and when I looped around again I stopped and imagined that all the streaks of light trailing the comet were angels scurrying back through the window like kids trying to sneak back into the house past curfew.

Angels, spirits, ghosts, and the supernatural were all things that I had thought about a lot since the time of Lisa's death, much more than I had ever thought about them before. All the conversations with the kids regarding their mom being an angel and the books that I would read to them that spoke of angels made me really confront whether I truly believed in that type of stuff or not. There is a big part of me that really wants to believe that there are angels (or something like them) out there watching over us, keeping us safe. This is a useful and comforting concept, especially for kids, to have in the back pocket. For me it was similar to a child's belief in Santa Claus until a series of unexplainable things happened that made me start to seriously consider the possibility of something more real than a chubby elf in a red suit, flying around in a magic sleigh.

It's difficult to say exactly when the weird stuff started happening, because I wasn't looking for it and may have missed some things. It was shortly after Lisa's death when I noticed the first of many bizarre things. For the most part, they were not earth-shattering or haunting. Nothing like what was portrayed in "Poltergeist," but there were definitely some episodes that were kind of hard to explain away simply as coincidences. The common theme through most of the weird incidents was electricity, such as televisions mysteriously turning on in the middle of the night.

The electrical disturbances began slowly and then picked up in both frequency and intensity. It started with streetlights. When I went out for my inaugural middle of the night run, I felt funny about leaving the kids in the house by themselves at 4 o'clock in the morning. Lisa would have had a fit if she knew I was doing this, but I really needed to run and this was the only time I could go without the hassle and expense of getting a babysitter. As I was running down a dark side street, one of the three streetlights popped and went out just as I ran underneath it. This made me jump. It was still a couple of hours before the lights should go out for daybreak as evidenced by the fact that none of the other lights on any of the other streets were out. So, I figured (like any rational person) that the bulb had just burned out. A couple of mornings later as I was running past the entrance to our neighborhood, the flood light that shone on the entrance sign sparked and went out. Yet another morning, running down one of the longer main streets next to our neighborhood, three street lights in a row went out as I ran past each one. These occurrences, because they had happened so close together, started to spook me a bit. What if this was Lisa's way of communicating to me that I had better get my ass back to the house and stop leaving her babies unattended like that? The eerie thing is that all these lights would be working fine the next morning. It was always a different one that went out, never the same one twice.

I know there is nothing really exciting about streetlights, but they started to go out all over the place, just about everywhere I went. The place where all the kids took gymnastics was just down the block from a little, run down cemetery. The first time we drove by the cemetery after Lisa died, Gaven pointed out the window and said "Look, that's where Mom is buried." Just as she was blurting out that interesting and erroneous observation, the lone light just above the gate at the cemetery's entrance went dark. I was already jumpy about these electrical episodes, and this one caught the attention of the kids. From that night on, that light would go off almost every week either as we were going to or coming back from gymnastics.

One Wednesday night, the kids and I were driving home from church after their choir practice and youth group meeting. We were about a mile from home when all the lights on both sides of the street for the last half of that block suddenly and simultaneously went out. Then as I turned the corner all the lights up to my next turn went out and this continued for the next four blocks through our neighborhood all the way to our cul-de-sac. The final light that went out was the lone light at the end of our street that was right in front of our house. It went out as we pulled into our driveway and never came back on. I just drove all the way home with my mouth hanging open watching the lights disappearing and wondering what in the heck was going on.

Every once in awhile, when I had an opportunity to run during daylight, a streetlight would come on as I ran past. I wondered if she still had her days and nights mixed up.

On occasion, the level of electricity involved in these episodes was potentially harmful. Like the time when Lisa's good friend decided to separate from her husband, and moved out of their beautiful home into a small, inexpensive apartment. Lisa never did care for her friend's husband and apparently applauded her bold move with a large clap of lightning that struck the house the night after she left him. It occurred to me that perhaps Lisa was either pissed off or being funny.

The uncommon incidents were not always electrical in nature. The kids and I had often thought that their mom, who was very musically inclined, was at times part of the wind directing the chimes to play pretty music. Sometimes when we spoke her name puffs of wind seemed to come out of nowhere and played the chimes like fingers running across the strings of a harp.

My dad said,
She plays a harp with
Strings made of sunbeams
From sunsets.

My dad said,
If she wants us to hear
The notes are shot down
To whistle thru the leaves
And make the birds sing.

My dad said,
If you close your eyes
You can feel her music
On your face and smell
It in the breath you take.

My dad said,
Sometimes when she visits
She plays the chimes with
Fingers of wind touching
Them like strings on a harp.

My dad said,
Sometimes when we can't sleep
She sings us a lullaby
Which closes our eyes and
Brings us sweet dreams.

My dad said,
When we feel like dancing
And no music is playing
It's her songs in our heart
That make our feet happy.

     I had noticed something else kind of amazing about the wind and the balloons that the kids let loose on their mom's behalf. Of all the balloons that these kids have let go (and there have been a bunch), not a single one has ever gotten snagged. They have always managed to clear all obstacles and make their way to the destination, heaven. Not one has ever drifted into a tree and popped, or got its string caught, and the kids have let balloons go from some pretty tight launching pads. Just when it appears that there is no way a balloon will be able to rise quickly enough to clear a tall pine tree, a gust comes along and shoots it straight up over the top, free to float unhindered until it's snatched up by their mom.

One event really sticks out in my mind. Gaven came out of the gymnastics facility after a friend's birthday party clutching her bag of party favors and a balloon. The building was tucked away pretty tightly in a thick grove of trees and because of a fairly strong breeze my scientific mind calculated that there would be no chance of a successful launch. "Dad, can I let my balloon go for Mom?" Gaven asked.

"Gaven, I really don't think the balloon will make it past all those trees because the wind is blowing too hard. Why don't you wait until we get home where there is a lot more room. I would hate for it to get stuck or pop on the branches. Don't you think that's smart?"

Trying to reason with a four-year old is like trying to reason with a puppy. "It will be okay, there is lots of room for a balloon," she said letting loose of the string. We stood in the parking lot watching it head straight for the trees. It would have needed a last second vertical hurricane to save it. It hit the very first tree. The balloon bounced back and forth among the lower fat

179

branches and wiggled its way out only to run into the next in an endless clump of trees. Somehow it dodged one tree completely and started to weave it's way, side to side, avoiding disaster after disaster, and just when it looked like it had a chance, it got wedged tightly between two branches. This was a determined little balloon. By now a small group of spectators from the party had gathered to cheer the balloon on. The wind seemed to pick up, and its string started moving back and forth violently like a salmon's tail as it tries to swim up a waterfall. If I hadn't known better, I would have sworn that I could hear it grunting. Then, just like the salmon as it leaps free from the water, the balloon took a leap, broke free from its captor and rose quickly above the other treetops. Gaven cheered along with the rest of the crowd, and I just stood there shaking my head.

I don't know what all this means, but maybe when I die I will somehow get to follow along with the people I cared about, even if just long enough to see them through any tough times that my death may have caused. When I was a kid about Samantha's age, I used to think that if I died I would still be able to see and hear everything through one of my brother's eyes and ears. Kind of like being inside his head without him knowing it. Maybe that's a weird thing for a child that age to be thinking, but after reading some of the stories my kids have written in school, I was probably fairly normal.

Maybe when I die I will be allowed to come and hang around earth, but in some other life form such as an animal, insect or even one of the forces of nature. Reincarnation as a particular form or force may be dependent on one's personality type or special talent. Heaven and hell (if there are such things) might consist of the circumstances of one's return to earth. If you were a good person you get to come back as something decent like an eagle, or if you are really sweet then maybe you come back as the scent of a flower. If you were selfish and whiney, then you might get to come back as a slug or a mosquito. Throughout Lisa's illness she was really angry, and that might explain why all this electrical stuff started happening. Electricity could be hazardous if she was a mean person, but she wasn't. She would never intentionally hurt anyone, which is a good thing for me. She would, however, get a kick out of scaring the shit out of someone.

If this scenario were true I have to wonder about the form I would take for my return to earth. If I could choose, it might be as some kamikaze microorganism that would help to stop the cow from eating everyone. If not that, then maybe I could just be a giant fly that could buzz around its face long enough to at least slow it down.

Do I believe in spirits and angels? No one has disproved their existence to me, and I have seen and felt some remarkable things, so why not? I like to think they are out there somewhere, and I continue to look for signs that they do exist. I am frequently reminded of the night my son Ben went running outside to see if he could catch a glimpse of his mom's spirit rising just after she passed away. Children, because of their open-minded and uncontaminated beliefs, are more likely to believe in angels, spirits, and Santa Claus. Maybe those qualities are necessary to actually see or feel them.

Animals are also thought to have a sixth sense that picks up on supernatural activity. Dusty slept in the garage at night, which is where she was the night Lisa died. As a multitude of people came in and out of my house that evening, Dusty didn't move, didn't make a sound. But when they carried Lisa's body out of the house, Dusty started barking and didn't stop until they put Lisa in the truck and drove off. At the time it gave me giant goose bumps, and prompted a discussion with my dad, George and myself about the dog's sixth sense theory. Lisa was not a dog fan. She was more of the cat type, and liked to take cheap shots at how dumb dogs were, but she was also the one that fed Dusty, took her to the vet, and looked the hardest for her when she got frightened by lightening and ran away. They were bonded even if she would never admit it. Maybe Dusty started barking because she sensed that the person who gave her food was gone and was worried that no one would take care of her. A valid concern, even coming from a dog. Dusty may have been trying to tell me to get ready for some weird stuff. She'll, "roofff" be, "rooff" back, "roooff-roooff."

Because I was looking for it, I saw signs of angelic activity in things that at other times in my life may not have suggested angels to me. It would be like two different people staring at the same cloud. ("Doesn't that cloud look like an angel?"

"Are you crazy? That cloud looks like a hump back whale.") Just after the only snow of one entire winter, the kids and I spent the day building snowmen and making snow angels. They filled up a good portion of the backyard with their little winged body prints. After we all came inside to warm-up, a gentle southerly wind came up and warmed the air. In the late evening I looked out of my second story window to the place in the backyard where the kids had made their snow angels and I noticed that they were gone. The air had warmed just enough to melt those spots snuggly into the ground. What was left was one huge, perfectly shaped angel, which somehow was the unintended and trans-formed some of our many smaller angels. It was awesome, com-plete with flowing hair, halo and a set of wings that took up most of the back yard. The next morning I woke just as it was starting to get light and I quickly went to the window to see our angel. To my disappointment the warmth of the night had released the angel from it's frozen canvas and her picture was gone.

Confronting the Cow

Warm snow falling on her soul
Juicy flakes larger than the wide-eyed sockets
Outstretched tongues nourished
By the angelic floating tear drops
Spirited purposefully to earth.
She rests on the grass
Surrounded by snow in and out.
Her heart melts at the edges,
No crystals survive the landing.
Wings spread ready for flight
Escaping quietly under cover of night.
Her image remained like an unmade bed
And will stay forever inside their heads.

Escape In the Night

One by one I gently scooped up each sleeping child. As quickly as possible I carried them down the stairs, out the front door, and into the van. It was 2:30 a.m. and cold, even for the middle of March. I had started the van earlier and cranked up the heater so the shock of the cold would not wake them. It had only been a couple of short hours since I finished packing their bags. Each of them was allowed one large duffel bag to pack their clothes and any personal items as long as it fit in the bag. Finally, at 12:30 a.m., I had closed the door on the rented U-haul trailer and laid down on my bed for a short catnap. The medium sized trailer was packed full with bicycles, file cabinets, computers and a few other miscellaneous necessities. This was a difficult packing job because we only had room for two weeks worth of stuff, even though for all practical purposes we would be gone forever. As we pulled out of the driveway I looked back at the four sleeping babies. It felt like I had just kidnapped someone's children (actually grandchildren), and was trying to escape undetected in the middle of the night.

185

Since the streetlight in front of our house still didn't work it was very dark, but the red tail light of the trailer allowed me to see the "For Sale" sign in the front yard as we drove away. We were moving to North Carolina.

My job offer, much to the benefit of my blood pressure, finally became official in early February. Originally I was hoping to work it out so that I could wait until the kids were out of school before starting this new job. I thought that waiting to move until summer would be easier on the kids, and would also give me adequate time to sell my house. But by the time the offer came I was so eager to leave that I agreed to a start date that was only six weeks away. This obviously was not enough time to sell my house, buy a new house, pack all of our belongings and move to North Carolina. My back up plan was to gather up a few of our necessities, a couple weeks worth of clothes, drive to North Carolina and move in with my brother until my house sold. My brother and his wife also have four kids (three girls and a boy) whose ages stagger perfectly in between the ages of my kids. Eight truly will be enough.

The job offer hadn't come easy, and even though I was qualified for the position I felt the deciding factors were a combination of George's letter of recommendation and my use of Super Cow Man's powers of persuasion. It would be difficult to turn down a man who had just lost his wife to cancer, had four little kids to take care of, and who desperately needed to start a new life. Plus, I was genuinely excited about working for a medical institution because of the possibility of helping sick people. Armed with a glorifying letter from an employee of God in one hand and a picture of my angelic kids in the other hand, it had to have been almost impossible to turn me down. In years past I would have never played up to people's emotions to get anything, and I wasn't really doing so on purpose. But it had become a built-in survival mechanism that kicked in automatically. I felt like I had to have that job, and I was ready to do whatever it took to get it. As hard as it was finding this job, it still was infinitely easier than telling Lisa's parents that I had accepted a new position and would be moving with the kids to North Carolina in six weeks.

I walked into their family room where they were reading the Sunday paper and sat down on the sofa across from them. They were immediately suspicious because I rarely (if ever) sat long enough to read the paper or engage in casual conversation. For about the millionth time I was second-guessing myself about my decision not to talk to them from the beginning about my desires to move. If only I had applied the same up front communication with them that I had been adhering to with the kids this moment would have been a lot less painful. Typically when we went to their house after church I always stayed outside or down in the basement playing with the kids. I'm just not a sit down and chat kind of guy, especially when my four kids are running loose at someone else's house. Somehow I couldn't help but feel responsible for their actions. Granted they are always perfect angels and require no supervision but there is still that chance of an accident. "How did that window get broken?"

"What window?"

"The window with the golf club sticking through it."

"Oh, that one. We don't know, it was like that."

I sat on the sofa with my arms spread across the back and my legs crossed trying to look like my stomach wasn't tied up in knots. We talked about the weather and the local basketball teams then I took a deep breath, which they had to have heard. I inched out to the end of the high dive, checked the wind conditions, counted to three and jumped. Instead of yelling "Geronimooooooo," I yelled "we're going to mooooove," splat; a belly flop.

"We kind of figured you would have to do this someday," was all they said. Then they sat there silently on their favorite chairs, shaking their heads up and down and grinning. They weren't grinning because they were happy about us leaving, they were grinning because their intuitions had been correct. They were those "Yep, we were right" kind of smiles which made me feel slightly embarrassed. Then it was up to me to fill the silence with the details, which only took a few minutes. Still, they sat there quietly, just staring and nodding at me. So I repeated the details again, first backwards, then sideways, then in Chinese, and finally I got up and went outside to scream. It was like hitting myself in the thumb with a hammer over and over again and holding all the painful yells inside until I could run way up on top of the farthest hill and let it all out. In truth, there really wasn't a whole lot that they could say. They are smart folks, and they picked up on the fact that I said I had accepted a job and not that I was thinking about accepting a job. The fact that I had not consulted with them prior to this announcement made them realize that I had made up my mind and there wasn't much that they could say to make me reconsider, and they didn't try. "We understand that you need to do what you think is best for yourself and the kids. We really hate to see you leave, but we totally support any decision you make and if there is anything we can do to help, we will."

While they were telling me this I just sat there and smiled because I had prayed that this is what they would say and was relieved when they did. "Thanks, you don't know how much that means to me. I about gave myself ulcers worrying about how you guys would take this decision. It was not taken lightly, let me assure you. But right now it is something that I have to do."

At that time I believed that our leaving would allow Lisa's family a chance to catch their breath and focus their efforts on some other important things that had been put on the back burner for two years. The rest of Lisa's family had their own lives outside of her sickness that they could now concentrate on more fully. Lisa's sister was pregnant with her first child, and with us gone her parents could devote a lot of positive energy to the birth of this new baby. This had to have been a huge emotional swing, going from the heartache of sickness and death to the joys of birth and new life. Hopefully it helped take the edge off of the sorrow they were experiencing. We had been such hogs of people's time; it felt good seeing others getting their overdue share of positive attention.

After I told Lisa's parents my plans we didn't talk about it much further. They seemed more relaxed than I had seen them for a long time. They continued coming over to watch the kids whenever I had gaps in my babysitter and day care coverage and Lisa's dad started coming over to the house when I was at work to do little odd jobs that would help make it more saleable. Their supportive attitude lifted a tremendous burden from my guilt-ridden conscience. I realized how fortunate I was to be a part of their family.

Those six weeks went by very quickly, as there were many things to accomplish before we left town. Trying to sell the house was my main concern, which meant keeping it clean 24 hours a day. The only way to keep the house clean was to keep the walking dirt balls out of there, which was not easy to do. We ate at McDonalds a lot so I didn't have to clean the kitchen as often.

Lisa's parents frequently had us over for dinner, which helped a bunch and also reminded the kids that not all meals came in sacks with a toy. I had also optimistically started packing boxes, which slowly removed some unneeded clutter.

One of the more disappointing and anti-climatic things that happened during those six weeks was my resignation. I had spent the last 15 years of my life working for this company and put in more waking hours there than I had at home. This was also the company that had stood by me and was so patient with me during the past two years as we battled Lisa's illness. You would think that there would have been a large farewell party on my last day, complete with handshakes, speeches filled with bad jokes and unwanted gifts from my long-time cohorts. But because I had moved so many times in the past few years this scene never materialized. The people I was working with at the end barely knew me. In fact many of them even seemed to be afraid of me.

My boss organized a small luncheon and probably made it mandatory that the people in her group attend. I drove myself to the restaurant and was placed conspicuously at the head of a large table. Everyone had signed a card wishing me well. It was such an uncomfortable and awkward situation that I was actually one of the first people to leave.

I went back to the office one last time to turn in my badge and gather up the few personal belongings from my desk, which consisted of some pictures of the kids, a permanently discolored coffee mug and a super ball. As I walked out the front gate for the very last time carrying my small box of stuff, there was a hollow and empty feeling in my stomach. It was hard to believe that this was how my career at this company would end. Was this all the last 15 years amounted to, a lunch with strangers and a box of trinkets? It was a good indication that my decision to move on was the right thing to do.

In a way this was the same feeling I had when we finally left town. There was no big send-off or party. I had only one or two good friends that I would actually miss. There was a small gathering of people at Lisa's parents the night before we departed which was primarily family and a few of the neighbors that we had met since moving back to Kansas. We couldn't stay too long because I still had to pack all the kids' bags and get them ready to leave their house forever. There was one last round of hugs as Lisa's parents tried to get an imprint of their grandchildren that would stick in their minds until they saw them again. When it was time to leave I hoisted Gaven up to my shoulders as we had done many times before, and walked back home. Then, with just a small portion of our worldly possessions, we snuck out of town under the cover of darkness and we were gone. Poof.

The expressionless lady in the little booth handed me the ticket for the toll. The green light flashed, the striped arm lifted up, and we were on our way to our new home. I looked back in my rear view mirror and saw four flush-lipped babies and smelled one dirty dog, all sleeping peacefully. Not once did my kids (or the dog) ever question my decision to move. When I first asked them what they thought about the possibility of moving to the same place where their cousins lived, they got genuinely excited and begged to move. Now they slept with necks twisted in abnormal positions, trusting me so completely, knowing that I would never do anything that would be bad for them. That definitely made it easier to get them into the car. I only wished that I had their faith in what I was doing. Nonetheless, we were on the road. Our hotel reservation for that coming night was in Nashville, which was over 800 miles away.

Because of the long distance I needed to travel on that first day, having them sleep for at least the first five hours was critical to my travel plans. If they had sensed my anxiety they would have been unable to sleep so soundly. Maybe Ben did sense something, because not more than 15 miles down the highway, his little head started gyrating back and forth, and his hand found its way to his crotch. A moment later I heard a moan, which I ignored and hoped would go away. "I need to go to the bathroom." I turned the music up a bit and hoped that he would just fall back asleep and forget about his bodily functions for awhile. "I need to go to the bathroom," he said again with a little more urgency.

"God Ben, can't you wait for a little while? We just got started."

"No Dad, I got to go real bad."

I pulled off on the shoulder and opened the big sliding side door of the plum colored mini-van and Ben stood there, in the van, peeing on the highway. It's times like these that make me feel proud to be a male. But alas, the van door was an open invitation for the wicked wind of the west as it whipped in and woke all the sleeping munchkins. "Are we almost there yet?"

"How much farther do we have to go?"

"I'm hungry."

"I have to go to the bathroom."

It took us two days to finish the 1300 mile trip which went very smoothly, with the exception of a brief period in Nashville when some might say I got lost as I tried to find the hotel. It was rush hour and I kept driving around the same loop over and over thinking it would somehow miraculously appear. My kids all started yelling at me because they were hungry and had been in the car for 15 straight hours. "Dad, are you lost?"

"Don't you know how to get there? Just look at the map."

"Why don't you stop and ask someone like Mom always did?"

"I have to go to the bathroom."

My butt was sore, I was starving, and I was in no mood

for getting grilled from a bunch of little kids. "The next time someone opens their mouth I'm going to stop the car and let all of you walk to North Carolina!" That sure sounded like something my dad used to yell at us back when we took those long, cross country family vacations.

When we finally found the hotel the kids wisely cheered "Hurray for Dad!"

"Dad's the greatest driver in the world."

"Yeah Dad, you're the best hotel finder ever."

"Okay, that's enough. Do you guys want a straw with that," I said making a sucking noise that so that they knew that I was on to their obvious attempts to butter me up after I had been so mad at them. "Maybe if you keep talking like that you might get some supper."

The kids took that as some kind of a challenge and with windows rolled down we pulled into the parking lot with a well-rehearsed chorus, "Dad's number one. Dad's number one. Dad's number one."

"I'm number one," I chanted as held up my index finger and waved as we drove by a startled elderly couple and their dog.

The second day of travel was much easier, mainly because it was only 500 miles rather than the 800 miles we had traveled the first day. As we drove by the "Welcome to North Carolina" sign the kids', excitement grew. It was good to see them so happy. As the miles clicked off and we got closer to our final destination I started feeling apprehensive about the whole move. New job, new schools, living with my brother, leaving the security of their grandparents, was I really doing the right thing?

By the time we turned onto my brother's street I was a nervous wreck. It didn't help matters any to drive through this upscale neighborhood in my down-scaled squeaky old van, piled high with junk, and pulling a trailer also filled with assorted junk. I felt like we were part of a traveling circus arriving at our show destination. Especially when we parked in front of his house and all these noisy short people and a mangy fat dog piled out of the van door. The neighbors were probably horrified. We had landed and I took a moment to exhale and pinch myself because I was having a real hard time believing that we were actually here to stay. That lasted for about a second and then the reality of the situation hit me as the sight of my brother, wife and four kids reminded me that the eleven of us were going to be living in the same house for some unknown amount of time. I was out of control, again.

The kids were so thrilled to see their cousins as they came running up to greet them. They all started screaming and doing cartwheels, then just that quick the whole pack ran inside the house to see where everyone was going to be sleeping. That night eight kids had dinner, eight kids had baths, and eight sets of clothes were laid out. My brother and I formed a mini assembly line as we mass produced eight brown sack lunches, which were placed neatly in the fridge ready for the next school day. I had completed the school registration paperwork on my last visit, and because of my sister-in-law's involvement at the school we were able to meet with the principal and hand pick which teachers we thought would be the best for Samantha and Emily. After the first day of school Samantha was in tears because her classroom was too chaotic and loosely run, and she felt lost. After a call to the principal Sam was in a different, more structured class and was all smiles from then on. That first day was also Emily's birthday, and one of her aunt's friends had gotten her a new dress and a special candy bouquet to wear to help her meet new kids. Emily felt very special. Ben and Gaven were still in pre-school and my sister-in-law, because of her high ranking in the Mommy Network, got them in this great school ahead of the many others who were already on the long waiting list. Car pools, play dates with other kids, all those important little things were all taken care of. She was a highly respected person in the area, and I got to reap the benefits of the years of hard work that it took to reach this high ranking. We were treated like royalty, which made the kids feel instantly welcome and made me feel like I had done the right thing in bringing them here.

The fact that everyone got along fantastically under these extreme circumstances was no accident. A lot of effort and personal sacrifice went into making sure that our stay under my brother's roof didn't turn into a bad memory. My brother and sister-in-law treated my kids as their own and never complained about us being there. All the extra laundry, the huge meals every night, making eight lunches before school, putting up with our dog, sharing their time, and I could go on and on. They did so much and wanted nothing in return but to see us do well. Their kids were equally amazing as they willingly shared their rooms, toys and even their mom (who was in big demand) without hesitation. An occasional squabble erupted over whose turn it was to play the video games on the computer but it was nothing that pulling the plug out of the wall wouldn't fix. They all became very good friends and it was heartwarming to watch. Everything seemed tolerable as long as they were all together, even when all eight of them had head lice at the same time and had to sleep with their hair dripping in olive oil while wearing big plastic bags over their head. It was so ridiculous, and because there were so many of them it was funny, almost.

These forces that brought our families together were born of intense sources that were not easy to deal with, but my brother and sister-in-law never backed away. The sacrifices they made as they put their lives on hold to help us will never be forgotten. In fact it will have made such a lasting impression on my kids that they will no doubt be proudly telling this story as an example of family togetherness to their children for years to come.

Initially, all I really cared about was that the kids were all right. My new job was decent, but it was still just a job that I needed to pay my bills. I didn't have a real life of my own yet. My brother was kind enough to hand me a suit from his closet and said, "Here, wear my life for a while until you get settled in and have time to find your own."

"Thanks Bro, let me try it on." Luckily we have always been about the same size and his suit fit pretty well, but it still felt borrowed. It would be a happy day when I could walk in wearing my own duds and return my brother's fresh from the cleaners.

After a month or so we had gotten settled into kind of a routine, which meant it was time for me to start feeling anxious. I also felt a slight twinge of anxiousness from my brother. Even though everyone had adapted to this arrangement, we all knew that this could not continue indefinitely. My brother's family needed their lives back and we needed to establish our own. The first and most crucial step was to get a house. This was complicated by the fact that my house in Kansas still had not sold, and there weren't any interested buyers at the time. But I couldn't wait any longer. I decided to go out on a limb and buy a house with the hopes that the one in Kansas would sell soon. Here I go again.

As it had in Kansas, it felt incredibly good to go looking for a house with the idea that I was actually going to buy it instead of just window-shopping. Finding the house was easy. There was a neighborhood just down the road from my brother's that was loaded with young families and was in the same school district. The tricky part was the financing. First I tried a traditional mortgage company, and they basically laughed at my situation. Fortunately my brother knew a guy who was, as he described, a little bit flaky, but specialized in creative financing. He came up with a plan. It wasn't too farfetched, but when I signed on the dotted line it felt like I had made a deal with the devil (which at the time would have been okay with me). The danger of this deal was that if my other house did not sell I would have to make double house payments, which I figured I could do for a couple of months before having to declare bankruptcy and live in a box.

Just before the final closing on my new house a small miracle happened. My real estate agent from Kansas called to present me with an offer on my house. Judging by the amount of the offer the people must have suspected that I was desperate. They were right and I took the offer even though I would lose a good chunk of change on the deal. In return, I received peace of mind that was worth every cent. I just kept telling myself that it was only money.

For the first time in years I started to feel in control. It had been such a helpless feeling having to rely so totally on Lisa's parents and then on my brother's family for just about everything. When I saw my brother mowing his yard it really hit me how badly I needed to be on my own. I had been trying to live their life. The more I did so the more I realized how much different I was from them, and how important it was that I started swimming around in my own fish bowl.

Moving. I swore that after this move I would never move again. I told my boss that I needed to take a few days off so I could go to Kansas, pack up my whole house on a dinosaur and ride it all the way back to North Carolina. Then unload and stack a bunch of boxes into my new garage forming a cozy set of high rise condominiums for roaches.

Before the kids and I made our great escape I had managed to pack the entire kitchen and most of the kids' closets into moving boxes. I also had gone through all of their toys to see what I felt they could live without, which in my moving mode was almost everything. I dedicated an entire Saturday afternoon to determining the fate of the truckloads of non-educational toys in our basement. Garbage bag after garbage bag I filled with all the "junk" that I had grown so tired of picking up every day. Almost all of it would never be missed and would never be asked for again. But if the kids were there watching me dispose of these treasures they would swear that each plastic car and naked Barbie was their most prized possession. Since I did not have a dump truck big enough for my quarry, it went into the trash so I could make room for Beanie Baby accessories.

When I arrived back in Kansas to gather our belongings

there was still a lot of work to do just to prepare items for loading onto the truck. I had quite a bit of help, so it went rather quickly. The hardest thing was trying to decide what stuff I really wanted to take and what stuff I was going to leave for the big going out of business sale that Lisa's dad offered to have for me after I had gone. Basically there were four categories. There was the 'keep' category, there was the 'Goodwill' category, there was the 'I need some cash' category, and the 'trash' category. At the time I was more inclined to throw stuff away than to keep it or sell it.

There was also the task of deciding what to do with Lisa's personal belongings. I had left everything in her closet pretty much untouched. Her family had an opportunity to take anything of hers that they wanted to keep, and the rest was left for me to contend with. I decided not to keep much, except for some things that I could give to the kids as they grew older. Then I placed her belongings in a large plastic container and sealed it up like a time capsule. The rest of her things either went to Goodwill or in the trash. It wasn't fun or easy, but was necessary and a part of moving forward that I could not delay any longer.

While I was in Kansas, I took the time to drive out to the cemetery. I knew that it would be a long time before I got back there so I thought it a good idea to take this opportunity for a visit. It was late morning on a weekday and I was the only living person for miles. When I approached her grave a black crow flew out of a nearby tree and spooked me a bit. I stood there for a moment while the scenes from the funeral came flooding back. Emily's balloon popping, my parents getting lost, me sweating like a pig, and the kids' balloons as they sailed high over the lake. Then I sat down on the ground next to the grave, closed my eyes and felt the wind blowing across my face. At that moment I realized that graves were really just a formal place to remember a loved one, kind of like a church is a formal place to pray. I don't have to be in a church to pray just like I don't have to be at Lisa's grave to remember her. This holds true for the kids as well. We may have left places and things behind but we packed up as many memories as our hearts could carry.

Finally I was ready to load the truck. The first truck I picked up from the rental place was a nice new one and best of all, was an automatic. Of course this was too good to be true, for as I was driving it on the expressway home I noticed it acted funny whenever I got going over 50 miles per hour. I had to take it back. They only had one other truck in the lot that was big enough, but it was much older and was a stick shift. I was making beautiful gear grinding music as I left the parking lot and could only imagine the foot stomping tunes I would play as I ground my way through the mountains. Good thing it was a rental.

The last two items to go on the truck were my picnic table and lawn mower. Lisa's dad had been mowing my lawn for me while I was gone. Thirteen hundred miles was just a little bit too far to travel to cut the grass every week so I had to relinquish control of my yard. Ouch! It was going to be good to mow my new yard. In my head there would be a big ribbon cutting ceremony with some guy over the loud speaker saying "Gentleman, start your lawn mower."

The truck was full, and I had to slam the door quickly to keep stuff from falling out. Who needs professionals? I was ready to go. Lisa's parents and my brother-in-law, who had all helped load the truck, had already left for home. There would be no champagne-breaking bon voyages as the Titanic prepared to shove off. Then, for the very last time, I pulled out of my driveway and with one last glance in the rear view mirror I saw the 'For Sale' sign, but this time it also said "Sold."

With my elbow hanging out the window I headed down the highway. It was the most relaxing and enjoyable three days that I could remember. Truly a sign of my times, that driving an old rental truck through the likes of Kansas and Arkansas was to me a vacation in paradise. The truck would only go 65 mph so there was no point in trying to hurry. Driving across Oklahoma, Arkansas and Tennessee the only radio stations I could pick up were Country & Western. I kind of enjoyed the truck driving tunes and I made sure they were playing loudly when I pulled into the truck stops to fill up with diesel as if to say, "Yeah, Bubba, I'm a trucker."

Driving through the winding roads in the Smoky Mountains was a bit unnerving at times, and after I cleared the steepest and windiest part I stopped to check my cargo. When I opened the door and looked inside I thought that someone had switched trucks with me. My neatly packed truck had been rearranged so much that I didn't recognize it at first. My lawn mower, which was packed last was now somewhere toward the front. For the rest of the trip I decided that it would be best not to look until I got home.

It was a big moment when I backed that prehistoric beast into our new driveway. My kids, my brother and his wife and kids were all there waiting, and watched as I backed into the basketball goal. While I was gone, my brother and sister-in-law painted bedrooms, put the kids' new beds up, stocked the kitchen with various necessities and put toilet paper in the bathrooms. The kids loved their house, and after we unloaded the truck in world record time, we all sat down and had dinner at our familiar kitchen table. We were home, and it felt great as I swam up and down the stairs of my new fish bowl.

After everyone had gone home and I had put my exhausted but happy kids to bed, I got busy and put my bed together. It had been a long five days, and I was proud of myself for getting to this point. Then, as I laid my tired head down for a relaxing first night's sleep I started thinking about the reality of the whole situation. There I was, alone, with four kids, in a new town, with new schools, a new job and two mortgages. I started having yet another panic attack. My heart started racing and as I looked up at the ceiling fan directly above me I noticed that it had started going faster and faster until it sounded like a helicopter coming in for a landing. Just when it seemed as though the blades would go flying off, and my heart would jump out of my body, the fan started to slow down. It went slower and slower, and as it did so did the rate of the pounding in my chest. Finally both the fan and my heart were going very slowly, almost in rhythm, and I fell asleep.

Grandpa Duck

My kitchen had been painted by the shadow gray brush of early dawn and covered me with a thick double coat as I sat on the bench at my kitchen table. In my hand was another Race For The Cure entry form and with it came a sadness the likes of which I had not experienced for a long time. A tear welled up in my eye, catching me totally off guard. Crying was not one of my more well-known personality characteristics.

It had only been a couple of weeks since we had moved into our new house, and as I read through the race form I thought back on the previous two races we had participated in. The first one was after Lisa had gone into remission and I had allowed myself to slip back into a state of being semi fat, dumb and happy. The race ended with Lisa and the kids crossing the finish line, hand-in-hand, with a false hope of victory. The second race was after she died and the kids, with their undaunted and untainted attitudes, carried me through that extremely difficult time. What would this next race bring? Sometimes I wonder if it wouldn't be better to put these

207

races behind us. Why drag us through that again and again? Wouldn't it be easier and less painful to just send in a donation instead of rubbing salt into this deep wound and dredging up all those memories? 'Memories' is the key word here. That's exactly why we run the race. The sign that the kids and I had pinned on our backs read, "In Loving Memory of Mom," or "Lisa." She worried that we would someday forget her, and this race is just one of the many ways to make sure that we don't. She had good reason to worry because people are often rather quickly lost to time. In fact, it had almost happened to someone in my own family and I didn't even know it.

It had been a little over a year since Lisa was diagnosed, and she was in remission. We were up visiting my parents, who had retired on a lake in Northern Wisconsin. Whenever I go there I am reminded that my dad and brothers are true fishing fanatics. They never could understand why I didn't enjoy fishing as much as they did. Year after year I endured our family fishing vacations without complaining, but it was obvious that my heart was not in it. I was even made fun of for not loving to fish. For this reason I'm sure it was a shock to my father when he half-heartedly asked me if I wanted to go out for a short fish and I said "okay."

We loaded up the big red boat with all the necessary fishing gear, which included a small cooler of beer. How bad could this be? We had been out on the lake for over an hour without a bite. We kept moving from "hot spot" to "hot spot." My dad's commentary on each location kept a running dialogue going. "Last week I caught an undersized musky right about here."

"Oh really? I guess you had to throw it back."

Zoom. Over to the next spot we flew. "A few weeks ago your brother had a real nice strike right off the edge of that rock bar."

"Do you think it was a keeper?" I asked as I made the expected cast to the edge of the rock bar as if that same fish would still be there.

"Yeah, could have been. Well that's long enough here. If they don't hit right away we probably won't see any action." Zoom, to the next spot.

"Two years ago I had a real lunker follow my Bobbie bait right up to the boat."

"Man, I can't believe that fish didn't want to bite all those hooks," I said with a sarcasm that went unnoticed.

This familiar repertoire of my dad's was like background music to the sound of the waves slapping the side of the boat. It was actually quite relaxing, which was a sensation I had rarely experienced over the previous year. I honestly thought that if either one of us were to catch a fish it would spoil the peacefulness and probably get my dad's blood flowing enough to make him want to fish more aggressively. If anyone can actually fish aggressively, it would be my dad.

As I was standing there in the boat, casting my lure here and there hoping that the fish wouldn't like it, my dad spoke as he sent his lure whizzing out into the water. What he said made me sit down and grab a beer out of the cooler.

John Joseph was born in the winter of 1902 in a small Yugoslavian town. His parents were poor and the conditions under which his mother gave birth were not very good. Not long after he was born, his mother took ill and died. He was only an infant and never had the opportunity to know her.

John's father was devastated by the loss of his young wife and blamed himself and the State for not being able to provide a better existence for his family. He had heard stories of fabulous riches in America that were there for the taking, and he decided to go. In hopes of making a better life for his family, John's father left his young son with his grandma and headed out for this Land of Opportunity. After he found his fortune he would send for his family.

In 1904, as promised, he sent money for his family to get on a boat to come to the United States. John and his grandmother survived the rough voyage across the ocean, and his father met them on the shores of their new homeland. When they arrived, they were surprised to be greeted by not only his father, but by his new stepmother. The other surprise was that the wealth that was dreamed about had never materialized. The living conditions were not much better than they had been in Yugoslavia, but at least the family was back together. And now John had a mom to help take care of him.

John was a cute and happy little boy, but because of the hard times he was forced to wear some really large boots. When he was 7 or 8 years old his dad would send him out very late at night to the stockyards in search for lumps of coal that might have fallen from the freight cars. After midnight, he would bundle up, and sneak out into the darkness, pulling his little wagon. He had strict orders from his father not to come home until his wagon was full. Unfortunately, little John was not the only one out at the stockyards looking for the precious coal that was needed to heat the home and cook the food. Sometimes grown men would see him and take the coal he had loaded in his wagon. He would fight as hard as he could but they were too big and desperate. Tired and bruised, his search for coal would have to start over.

John had an opportunity to go to school, which he did up until the eighth grade. But because they were so poor, his dad decided that John's time would be better spent working. John had to quit school and work. Every penny he made had to be given to his father to help support the family.

The disillusionment of working so hard and never getting to spend any of the money he earned led him to run away from home to find work out on one of the farms. He was in his early teens when he stowed away on a farming wagon that took him safely out of town. He worked the whole summer in the nearby fields, saving every dime he made with the thought that when he went back to town after harvest was over he would take his money and buy himself some decent clothes that actually fit and weren't full of holes.

Summer ended and John went back home, but before he had a chance to figure out what to spend his life savings on his dad had found where he had stashed his money and had taken it. If that wasn't bad enough, his dad gave him a good beating for running off and trying to keep money that belonged to the family.

A year later John ran off again and got a job as a cook at a lumberjack camp up in the forests of Northern Wisconsin. He had never really cooked before, but he quickly learned and found that as long as the portions were large the hungry lumberjacks were happy. This time John wisely sent a sizable percentage of his earnings home for the family, which appeased his father.

John's sister wrote him a letter telling him that their father could get him a good job at the tool and die factory. She missed her brother and begged him to come back home. John missed his family too and decided to come back to town and take the job at the factory, but as soon as he was old enough he moved out of the house to live on his own. The factory job didn't make him rich but it provided a lot more money than he had ever had, and for the first time in his life he could spend it how he chose. He bought himself some new clothes and had some money to go bowling and hang out with his buddies down at the pool hall. He was a good kid, and even though he was no longer obligated he still sent some of his earnings to his parents. John continued to send his parents money until he got married and started having children of his own.

When John and Laura got married they were both in their twenties. Laura was a friendly girl, with beautiful skin and a warm heart, and everyone liked being around her. Together they had three children, two boys and the youngest a girl. It's expensive to raise a family, so even though John's job was decent and steady they still could not afford many luxuries. They did not have showers or bathtubs, so Laura would heat water on the wood stove and pour it into a large metal tub for the children's baths.

They lived in an old blue-collar neighborhood in Milwaukee, and were close to many of John's cousins and his sister. Compared to what John had been used to as a child, life for him now was very good. He had a steady job, a wife whom he adored, three beautiful children, family and friends nearby, and he got to fish, bowl and shoot pool with his buddies.

Then one day, when John came home from work, Laura showed him a sore that had developed on one of her breasts. She was a bit concerned because she didn't know what had caused it.

They kept a close watch on the sore thinking it to be some kind of skin rash and hoped that it would go away. But instead of getting smaller it proceeded to grow larger, so they decided that they should have a doctor look at it. The doctor examined her and concluded that it was indeed some form of skin irritation and prescribed a medicated ointment to be applied directly to the skin. Relieved, they went home and started treating the sore as prescribed, but it didn't work. In fact, by the time the ointment was gone it appeared to be making the sore on her breast even worse, so they went back to the doctor for a second look. This time the doctor did a complete exam and ran some tests. The results of the tests showed that Laura had breast cancer.

In those days there was not much known about breast cancer and there were virtually no available treatments. Because so little was known about this disease, people felt uncomfortable talking about it. Breast cancer was definitely not something that John would start tossing around with his buddies at the pool hall. The difficulties that adults had in dealing with cancer made it even worse for the kids as they were told nothing.

The cancer was slow but steady, and they managed to keep it concealed for over a year. The discomfort Laura was feeling in the beginning eventually intensified to the point where the basic pain relievers were no longer helping. The cancer had spread into her shoulders and it got to where she could no longer pick up her little daughter without grimacing. Eventually she couldn't pick her up at all.

Finally her symptoms were so noticeable that they could no longer keep the truth from the family. But still the word "cancer" was whispered around the children, so all they knew was that their mom was very sick.

The pain continued to get worse, and it finally reached a point where the only way to keep her remotely comfortable was with morphine. John was forced to come home from work and give her the injections himself. If he couldn't get home from work on time, his sister Bubbles would walk over and sit with Laura until he could get there. One time, Bubbles was walking to John's house and was still over a block away when she heard Laura screaming from the pain. Bubbles ran the rest of the way to try to help her, but the only thing that could help Laura was the morphine. Laura was writhing in such pain that when John finally got home with the medicine it was almost impossible to hold her steady long enough to give her the injection. She was so wild that when John did inject the needle it broke off in her arm. Their oldest son, John Jr., who was only eight, stood there and watched as his dad frantically tried to remove the needle from his screaming mother's arm. Finally, the morphine took over and she calmed down and slept.

The kids were not allowed to play in the house or have any friends over. They walked on eggshells around their mother who stayed covered up by blankets in her rocking chair. No longer could she walk with them to the drugstore for a piece of candy or come upstairs to tuck them in at night. After school the kids usually went over to their cousin's house until their dad came home from work. John said very little to his kids about their mother's condition. Laura wanted desperately to talk to her children, but she was so doped up that even if she wasn't asleep she found it almost impossible to speak sensibly.

Every night, after he put the kids to bed, John would sit with his bride and hold her hands and tell her the latest joke he had heard at work that day. Some nights she would sleep and some nights she sat awake speaking to people who were not there. He stayed up with her of course, patiently playing the many different characters in her make-believe dramas.

This went on for what seemed like an eternity. This strong, tall man in his thirties started to show signs of the strain and became more withdrawn. His focus narrowed as Laura's health deteriorated. The children became spectators and stood in the shadows as they watched their mother slowly disappear.

One night, the kids were in bed and John was sitting with Laura, holding her hands as always. Even though she was asleep, John noticed a change. Her breathing started to slow down and it continued to slow into the night. Finally, while John still had hold of her hands, she stopped breathing, and the two years of suffering was over. John laid his head down on her chest and wept.

To the children the funeral was a blur. They huddled around their aunt as their father cried uncontrollably. It was hard for them to watch their father, the rock that they lived on, crumble before them. Fear of what was going to happen to them now that their mother was gone raced through their young minds. All they knew was that at least they had each other.

John was a proud man, so it was with difficulty that he made the decision to have his daughter, his baby girl, live with his sister. He knew that this would be a better environment for her, realizing that she needed to be around someone better equipped to handle the needs of a little girl.

He was grateful for the help but it saddened him every day as he thought about his daughter walking to kindergarten with her uncle instead of with her mother. His boys, on the other hand, would be fine and would learn to take care of themselves. Once a week he would walk them up to the local natatorium where they would use the shower facilities. Boys just didn't need as much maintenance as did girls. Put them in a pair of jeans, a tee shirt, and run a comb through their hair and they were ready for anything.

For months John worked obsessively to keep up with the cooking, cleaning, and laundry while at the same time managing to go to his full-time job. Social workers would stop by from time to time to see how he was getting along. They were impressed with how clean and tidy he kept his house. They even remarked that his house was cleaner than the houses that had both a man and a woman living there.

Staying busy was good therapy and helped him keep his mind off of his sorrow. Sometimes staying busy wasn't enough and the pain got to be too much, even for him. Late one afternoon, John Jr. heard screaming coming from the kitchen. He walked to the doorway to find his father down on his hands and knees, pounding on the floor with his fists and yelling, "Why me, why me!" This frightened Johnny enough that he went next door to get his uncle who literally had to pull John up off the floor by the shirt and slap him in the face before he would stop.

Still the world kept spinning, and for six months John continued to pull this double duty of going to work and doing all the household chores. Then one day, while doing a load of whites at the Laundromat, he met Mary. Mary was quickly taken by this handsome man, as there was something especially appealing about a man who knew how to do the laundry. Mary and John began dating. Soon Mary started coming over to the house to help with the cooking and taking care of the boys. Mary and her daughter from a previous marriage both felt very comfortable around John and his children. The gloom that covered his house started to lift as John felt himself starting to fall in love again. A year later John and

Mary were married. Now his daughter, who had continued to stay with his sister, could come back home to live. John smiled. John's family was again complete.

Still John refused to talk about Laura, partly out of respect for his new wife, but mainly because it still was too painful. Mary tried her best to be supportive as John and his children continued to grieve the loss of Laura, but she found it very difficult living constantly in her shadow. Days, months, then years went by and the memory of Laura, the wife and mother, faded until she was almost completely erased from the children's chalkboards.

John and Mary worked hard to blend their two families and eventually their new family grew together as one. John's job was going well. The kids grew up loving their new mom and were happy to be together. They went on family vacations, which always seemed to involve fishing. The boys caught the fish and the girls cooked the fish.

Years passed and the kids grew up. John Jr. decided to go to college, even though it was against the will of his father who, like his father, thought young John's time would be better spent working. Stubbornness ran in his family, so while working full-time to pay his way, John Jr. successfully graduated in four years with a degree from the nearby University. Graduation day was a very proud moment for John Sr., for this was the first time anyone in his family had ever gone to college. He shed tears of pride. His family had come a long way since the days when he had to fight for coal.

John Jr. married his high school sweetheart, and they were soon on their way to raising a family of their own. They had five kids, four boys and finally a girl. They would all eventually grow up, find good jobs, get married, and have kids too. These were John Sr.'s great grandchildren. Whenever they saw him, Great Grandpa would quack at them like a duck and tickle their ribs. After a while the Great Grandkids started calling him Grandpa Duck.

Grandpa Duck was proud of this growing family he had started. They had endured some hardships that at the time seemed insurmountable, but no one ever gave up. Now he waddles around smoking his cigars, telling jokes and quacking like a duck at all the baby ducks.

"My mom died of breast cancer," he said as he automatically made another cast out into the lake.

I stared at my dad, 'John Jr.,' with my mouthing hanging open in utter disbelief. "Do you mean to tell me that your real mom died of breast cancer?"

"Yes, it's been so long now that about the only thing I can remember was my mom sitting in her chair all wrapped up in blankets and my dad coming home to give her shots," he said reflectively as he zinged another cast out into the lake.

I said nothing. The thought of my Grandpa giving his

wife injections sixty years ago really hit home for me. Flashbacks of the hundreds of shots I had given to Lisa over the past year played uncontrollably over and over in my head. The anxiety involved in pushing a needle into someone's flesh, especially if that someone (such as Lisa) was terrified of needles, should not be underestimated. My grandpa and I had not been well trained in the fine art of shot-giving and our wives had to suffer through our amateurism. Lisa endured the shots I had given her, but I almost think it was harder on me. Each time, the pressure of giving the shot was magnified by her fear stricken eyes and shaking hands. It was my job to make sure that the shots did not hurt and leave large, ugly bruises. I did not always succeed.

We didn't ask to be put in this spot, and our wives certainly did not deserve what happened to them. But there we were, and because we loved our families we would do without question whatever was needed of us. You would think, however, that based on the technological advances that we have seen over the last sixty years someone have would come up with a better way for certain medications to be given than putting needles in the hands of stressed-out amateurs.

Suddenly I could clearly see my grandpa, this funny and ageless old man, as a tall and strong young man of 36. He had three young kids, the oldest being my dad, who was only eight. I could see my grandpa coming home from work and gathering his children who were staying with some nearby relatives, and I could see my grandpa taking care of his very sick wife. I was certain that I could see him more clearly than anyone else, as the parallels between my grandpa's family and my family were stunning. Sixty years later, I was the tall, strong 36 year old man, coming home from work, gathering my four young children (the oldest also being only eight) who were also with nearby relatives, and taking care of my very sick wife.

My grandpa, Grandpa Duck, was suddenly transformed from this one-dimensional figurehead who I saw maybe once a year, to a person that I knew intimately and who knew me. There had been a sincerity in his voice when I spoke to him on the phone as he told me to "Hang in there," and that "Our prayers are with you." These were not just empty Hallmark card words, they were words from a man who had been there and understood what it was like, even though he had chosen to remain anonymous.

Now I could also see my dad at the age of eight, walking around his house quietly, through the room where his mother sat. The mother who was unable to take him to the corner store for a soda, and unable to go upstairs to tuck him in at night. My dad was like my kids and I could see it all. It made me sick to see how little had changed in the past sixty years. The cow had roamed the earth side by side with the dinosaurs, and it seems virtually indestructible and oblivious to time.

Grandpa Duck

Here I was, 36 years old, and this was the first time that I could remember my dad ever speaking of his birth mother, let alone how she had died. I knew that his real mom had died when he was a boy, but no one ever spoke of her or the circumstances. It made me wonder if I ever would have learned more about her if Lisa hadn't gotten cancer.

The reason I didn't know anything about this seemingly forgotten grandmother was because my grandpa never talked about her, so my dad never talked about her, so my mom never talked about her and we kids never knew to ask about her. It's amazing to me how effective the chain of command was in our family. There was this unwritten and unspoken law that we inherently obeyed without even asking. My hope, for Lisa's sake and for our children's, was to reverse this trend and make sure that her memory has an opportunity to make it to the next generation.

After his wife's funeral, my grandpa refused to speak of her for many years. Inevitably, memories of Laura faded. This was exactly what Lisa feared most, that she would be forgotten and become the mother that never existed. What had bothered me is that my grandmother was for all practical purposes extinct before my generation was even born. By the time I had come around, Grandpa Duck had been remarried for over thirty years and there was no mention of his first wife.

Why was it that my grandpa chose not to talk about this

person who was so important in his life and the lives of his children? Was it simply a characteristic of his generation not to talk about death, or was it some other product of the culture he grew up in? Quite possibly the biggest and simplest reason for his silence was that the loss of his wife, his best friend and mother to his children, was just too painful for him to talk about.

My brain started working real fast, and it played back comments that my dad had made to me about how impressed he had been with the way Lisa and I had been communicating with our kids. He could not believe how much they knew and how comfortable they were in talking about their mother and cancer. This undoubtedly made it easier for him to be around my kids, not having to walk on the same eggshells that he had walked on in his own house. It was obvious to me that things had been quite different for him when he was living through this as a child. Even though the similarities between what had happened to my grandfather and me are amazing, the differences in our cultures and the times in which we lived were so great that it makes comparing our experiences unrealistic and unfair.

In the end, we are not so much a product of what has happened to us over the course of our lives as much as we are a product of how we handled those happenings. Whether it is good fortune or tragedy, we have choices available as to how we react. It is these reactions that make each person different, and what is right for one person is not necessarily right for another. Because of our differing circumstances, my grandpa and I did not even have the same choices but we both did what we felt was right for us at the time. The way we communicated with our children regarding cancer, the approaches we used in dealing with death and funerals, and my ability to move my family to a new environment are all significant events that led us down different paths. Is one way better than another? I don't know. What I do know is that my grandpa's family turned out great and if I were handed that outcome for my family today I would take it and be happy.

In one important way, my approach will differ dramatically from Grandpa Duck's. His decision not to talk about his wife after she died may have helped him deal with his loss, but I think that it was unfortunate for his and Laura's children that they were not allowed the opportunity to develop lasting memories or images of their mother. My intentions are not to build a shrine but to merely incorporate the acknowledgment of Lisa's existence into normal, everyday life without obstructing the need to move on.

It was sad to see how far removed my dad's mother had become, and how few memories he now has. Is that just the way it is with young children? Is memory capacity so limited that even things as important as their mothers fade to almost total obscurity? When I try to remember what my mom or dad were like when I was eight, I draw a blank. I don't even remember pitching a no-hitter in a little league game. But I remember throwing up on my mom's lap as my parents were driving me to the hospital with pneumonia like it was yesterday. Memories seem to be somewhat uncontrollable. Will my efforts to develop lasting memories in my children be in vain?

A friend of mine who is about my age lost his sister to one of the cancer cows. She was only ten years old, and he was eight. He told me that he has very few real memories of her, and that most of what he can remember is the result of photographs that he has of her. This is unfortunately very consistent with what had almost immediately started happening with my kids.

It was maybe a year after their mom had died and I had asked an 'ist' from the hospice to come out and evaluate how my kids were doing. She asked each one of them what kinds of memories they had of their mom. As I listened in from my hiding place around the corner, I was saddened by how they struggled with this simple question. Gaven had chirped up, "I remember my mom took me to that one pizza place to eat and that she had no hair."

"She was a real good burper," blurted Ben as he proceeded to demonstrate how she sounded. There was no way he was going to let his little sister outdo him.

Even Emily and Samantha had a very hard time remembering any kind of real event involving their mom. But they each jumped up and got their own photo albums that their aunt had made for them, which were loaded with pictures of their mom. They could look at each of those pictures and tell some story about it. Still, it wasn't a real memory they were describing. They were simply reading the picture like they would read a book, but it was much better than nothing and some of those pictures might later trigger a memory.

Pictures, personal belongings, old letters or journals become the tangible things that keep loved ones around. But it is those intangible dreamlike thoughts and images that we really need to hang onto.

My dad's memories of what his mom was like before she was sick are very limited, but they are fond ones. Maybe the quality of memories is more important than the quantity. There is a sense that, more than detailed accounts, my dad had a feeling about his mother that is both warm and comforting. This feeling is better than a photograph and can't be put in a frame to collect dust on a shelf.

Maybe this is really the way it was meant to be, and this feeling is actually a chunk of his mom's spirit or soul that never goes away. The heart or soul of a person is the most important part. Surely we should not be judged or remembered for the body we lived in, but rather for who we were inside. Lisa often remarked how awful she looked and how afraid she was that the memory we would have of her would be one that included her ravaged physical appearance. Even though the kids enjoy looking at her healthy pictures, the real memory they hold of her is embedded deep inside of them, which is not so much physical as it is spiritual. When Samantha lies in bed some nights crying because she misses her mom, it's the warmth of her hug or the soothing sound of her voice that she can feel. When she closes her eyes she doesn't see a bald, crippled person with oxygen tubes in her nose, she feels a person who loved her more than her own life. She feels her mom, and this feeling hopefully will never fade.

Very few people live to be as old as my Grandpa Duck, who is now 98. He is one of a few remaining people who really knew Laura. Longevity has its price, and now Grandpa has to wonder who will be left to carry her memory forward after he is gone.

Ground Zero

I sat patiently and listened as each of the four women told her own tragic story. Each had lost a loved one within the past 18 months. The first woman had lost her father, the second's fiancee died suddenly, for the third it was her son, the fourth her sister, and finally there was me. The five of us had been asked to talk to a group of people who were in training to be bereavement counselors and who had learned about as much as they could from books. What they needed now were some real life examples of death, and the grieving that comes with it. These counselors in training needed to hear from the horse's mouth (or in my case the cow's mouth) what real grieving was all about instead of reading about it in a textbook or listening to a lecture. They needed to see the pain in our eyes and hear the anger in our voices. They also needed to get a feel for what makes us mad, and what we find helpful. These people, who are volunteers, are taking on a very difficult task in order to provide a much needed service, so when I was called and asked to help I eagerly accepted.

Even though I understood why they wanted me to be there, I couldn't help but think about what I was going to get out of this exercise. Maybe I would be able to get a sense for how well I was doing. In a way, I thought I might use these others as my grieving gauge and my wellness measuring stick. It had been well over two years since Lisa had died and I wanted to see how much progress I had made. As I listened and watched the others, I could hear and see the pain. One woman was finding it difficult to work because it no longer seemed important. The mother who had lost her son was angered when her good friend would talk to her casually about the activities of her own son. I heard and understood every word they were saying because I had been there, but at the same time I realized that I had moved past these places.

While I empathized with the others, I also felt a real sense of accomplishment. I constantly wanted to interrupt them to say that I understood. I wanted to jump up on the table like an overzealous preacher and tell them that I knew something, and that something was that with time the pain fades. It does get better. But I didn't interrupt them, because I also knew that at that moment they did not want to hear these trite "ist-isms," even from someone who had gone through a similar experience. It made these people angry, as it used to make me angry, when others tried to minimize their grief or dance around it by saying things like, "Oh, you are doing so well." Statements such as that, to someone who is grieving, have an effect similar to that achieved by saying, "Oh, you look so good" to a chemo patient. It can be very patronizing when coming from people who obviously don't get IT. Each person has to work through the grief in his or her own way, and at his or her own pace, as I did. So for me to have said to these others, "It gets better, it just takes time," would have been like a slap in the face. But hopefully, just by telling my story and explaining by example how I was doing, they would get a sense that I not only survived but that I was doing well without rubbing it in their face or trivializing their pain and anger. Maybe in me they could find and accept a glimmer of hope for themselves.

Even though much of my pain and anger had faded, my life was not like it used to be. My world had been turned upside down and looked very different. After Lisa died I was determined to reclaim my life and transform it from the needy existence that it had become. My goal was to be totally self-sufficient, and to allow all those wonderful people who had sacrificed so much on our behalf to have their lives back. I realized after many false starts that the only way for me to become self-sufficient was to basically start from Ground Zero.

What's Ground Zero? For me, Ground Zero was simply my kids and I doing the normal day-to-day things on our own. I decided that I simply would do everything for my family myself. Make lunches, get the kids to school, go to work, pick the kids up

231

from school, take the kids to dance and soccer, make dinner, clean the kitchen, help with homework, supervise baths, read bedtime stories, sign field trip permission slips, do the laundry, etc. In the midst of this unrealistic whirlwind I unwittingly and rather abruptly severed the lifelines to which I had been clinging. I shut the door on so many good, well-intentioned people. I put myself on an island, and my kids were ferryboats that gave me periodic access to the mainland. Any contact I had with people (other than those I was forced to see at work) was a result of my kids' activities. School functions, soccer games and swim meets became the social excursions off my island. They were "safe" activities, because I had my kids there to surround me and provide me with acceptable distractions when I needed to avoid other people.

Why had I become such an introvert? There were a few reasons. The first, which I have already mentioned, was my quest for self-sufficiency. Unfortunately I had come to associate any contact with my family and friends with personal weakness, so I stopped interacting with them. The second reason was that I was still in this protective mode which, over time, had become a part of my nature. I had become a mother duck. I strayed from my ducklings only when necessary, and it generally made me nervous and caused me to return very quickly to our nest.

The third reason for my hermit-like behavior was my total lack of social confidence. As soon as Lisa was diagnosed with cancer, my world shrank as I had no time for anything (or more importantly, anyone) that was not "necessary" to our family. Contact with my old friends dwindled down to nothing, and I consciously chose to shy away from new acquaintances even though I may have enjoyed their company. I knew there was no chance of sustaining any kind of real relationship. After I consistently turned down opportunities to play golf, or to join basketball teams, or to go out for a beer, people stopped inviting me. I lived this way for two solid, intense years. My life had been dressed in heavy layers of cowhide and tucked safely behind the walls of my house. If the cowhide wasn't enough insulation, I wrapped myself up in my children like security blankets.

It was hard to believe that I, who had always been a "life of the party" kind of guy, had become the insecure "wall flower." For so long when people would ask, "Hey Chris, how are you doing," my response was a run down on the status of each of the kids. "The kids are doing great," was one of my canned responses. Usually I didn't even mention myself, as in my mind my whole existence was measured by the health of my family.

Even in my isolation, Ground Zero was hard for me to find. I had to dig and keep digging, and for a while there did not appear to be a bottom. I was not even sure that I would recognize the bottom when I got there. Finally a realization came at about 3 o'clock one morning, when I woke up totally disoriented. I was still in my work clothes, the television was blaring, all the lights in the house were on and I was lying on my bed in the midst of a partially folded load of laundry. This wouldn't have been a big deal except that over the past couple of months this had happened to me at least six, maybe seven times. Like a good soldier I finished folding the clothes, turned off all the lights and checked on the kids. Then, as I crawled into bed it dawned on me how pathetic my personal life had become. The kids were doing well, which had been my primary goal, but waking up in the middle of the night fully dressed with my head resting on a pile of children's underwear was an indication that my life had become depressingly one dimensional. I had no friends and I had rather effectively extricated myself from my families. I had found Ground Zero.

At first it was very sobering, as I felt totally alone. Then as I thought about it more, I figured out that this was exactly where I wanted and needed to be. I found myself at the bottom of a very deep hole, but this time it was my hole. No longer was I at the mercy of so many uncontrollable factors. Even though I was in pretty bad shape, it was refreshing to realize that I had the power to do something about it. But this wasn't an exercise just for me. It was important for my kids that they have a "normally" functioning parent as a role model. I was not doing them any favors by performing all the chores around the house and sacrificing my entire life so that they could have it easier. In many regards they had been spoiled to help counteract the pain of losing their mother.

Now my task was to climb out of the hole in which I had placed myself. There were still some dangling vines and roots from the past that I attempted to use. Some were strong enough to sustain my weight while others either snapped or pulled out of the ground as I grabbed hold. It was clear that I was going to have to create some new footholds and give some of the existing ones a chance to strengthen before they would support me on my climb.

I couldn't help but think about one of my kids' books called "The Digging-est Dog." The main character, a dog named Duke, had spent a long time tied up in a pet shop and had forgotten how to interact with other dogs. He had never learned how to dig. Duke was overjoyed when Sammy Brown bought him, introduced him to other dogs, and most importantly taught him to dig. Duke was so excited that he went wild and dug up the whole town. Sammy and all the other dogs were angry with Duke for digging so thoughtlessly, and threatened to take him back to the pet shop. Duke couldn't bear the thought of going back to that life, so he started digging a hole to escape. He dug a hole so deep that he couldn't get out. Sammy and all the dogs looked down over the edge of the hole at helpless Duke and debated about whether to save him. Most of the dogs felt that Duke had dug his own hole and deserved his predicament. But Sammy Brown knew that Duke was a good dog and deserved another chance. Sammy convinced the others to help get Duke out of the hole. When Duke got out he was so grateful that he fixed all the damage his digging had done. From that point on Duke was very appreciative and grateful for his life and the second chance he was given. I realized that Duke and I had a lot in common.

Just months after Lisa died I remember hearing the news that Lance Armstrong, one of the world's best bike racers, had been eaten by the testicular cancer cow. At first there was a flurry of headline news regarding the status of his health. But the cancer cow was a slow moving beast, and our fast-paced society impatiently moved on. Soon the reports on Lance were reduced to sporadic one or two sentence updates on the back page of the newspaper's sports section. I suspected he was hidden away somewhere inside the cow. At the time I was very interested in this particular form of cancer, as I had started sensing some of this cow's symptoms in my own body. Due to my all too recent encounters with cancer, I was not about to let this go unchecked.

I promptly got on the web to find more information about this disease. As I was surfing I stumbled across a web site that appeared to belong to Lance Armstrong. It had a detailed account of his current health. Apparently the cancer was worse than originally diagnosed, and it had spread to his lungs and brain. He had surgery and was undergoing chemotherapy treatments. The "ists" gave him a 50/50 chance of survival.

The web site also provided a list of all the major symptoms of testicular cancer. The symptoms I had been experiencing were on the list, which scared the hell out of me. I immediately thought of my kids. Shaken, I continued to read the rest of the information until I got to the end of the web site. There, at the very bottom, set apart from the rest of the text was this simple message: "Good luck Chris." I freaked. This had to have been a message intended for a friend of Lance Armstrong's, but I wasn't about to try to find out. Instead, I got on the phone and scheduled an emergency physical (if there is such a thing).

My doctor was our family doctor. He knew all my kids and had known Lisa. He checked me out and sensed my nervousness, but he probably thought it was attributable to his rubber glove. I was relieved to find out that I was fine. "What about all those symptoms?" I asked.

"Those symptoms might be caused from having four kids whose heads are all about crotch high," he said unable to control his grin.

"Very funny, Doc. Make sure you put that in your report so the insurance company can have a laugh too."

Over the next couple of years I kind of lost track of Lance Armstrong's struggle (as I had enough of my own stuff to worry about) and had pretty much forgotten him until I saw that he was racing in the Tour de France. Of all sporting events, the Tour de

France is quite possibly the most grueling test of endurance (both physical and mental). Because of Lance's recent battle with cancer the race experts gave him very little chance of finishing, let alone winning, this event in which many of the participants drop out from sheer exhaustion. After 23 days and 2200 miles, Lance rode into Paris wearing the famed yellow jersey signifying victory. What the doctors, sports analysts, and the other competitors failed to understand was that Lance had successfully competed against the cow, which made pedaling over the Alps feel like riding across Kansas in comparison. Having watched Lisa struggle to get in shape to run/walk three miles and having personally competed in bike races, I can still only begin to appreciate the magnitude of what Lance Armstrong accomplished. He had been given a second chance and his triumph was a tremendous inspiration to me and countless others around the world. His accomplishment transcended the cancer context, and represented the boundlessness of the human spirit. It firmed my resolve to pick myself (and my family) up, dust off, and get back in the race.

Once again I was standing on top of a fog-covered mountain. But now the strong, hurricane-like winds had died down to a leaf-blowing breeze which tickled my scalp as it blew across my thinning, slightly gray, short bristly hair. The bottom of my long, hole riddled, T-shirt danced happily around the waist of my baggy blue jeans. There was a large wave of faded denim where the ends of my pant legs collided with my untied, grass stained tennis shoes. My feet were firmly planted on a small grassy area growing on the rock beneath me. I stood, with my eyes closed and face tilted slightly skyward as I welcomed the warm breeze. Then I opened my eyes and the dense fog had started to lift and suddenly for the first time in a very long while I could see my world. When the fog was gone I realized that I was not alone on top of a mountain. I was standing in my back yard with my own grass beneath my feet and my lawn mower singing sweetly before me. Gaven and Ben were on the swing set trying to yell over the noise of the mower, "Dad, can we have a super-duper push?" I saw Emily and Samantha ride by on their bikes as they were headed over to their friends' houses to play. I smelled the fresh cut grass and smiled.

A lot had happened to my family since the cow put an abrupt end to our fat, dumb and happy life. To say that my life had come full circle would imply that I was once again fat, dumb and happy, but that was not the case. The cow had left my kids and I face down on the side of the road, where we were left to pick ourselves up and put our lives back together. I had run too far and fast down the road to ever be "fat," and hopefully I had seen and experienced enough that my "Life IQ" had been permanently elevated above the "dumb" level. But what this brutal body and mind cross-training had given me was the capacity to recognize happiness and pursue it no matter how deep the hole or steep the climb.

The lessons learned from Lisa's determination to hold onto a life whose sweetness and preciousness all of a sudden had become crystal clear, and from the love that flowed from others when we needed it, would have been lost on me if I had continued to insulate myself from the world. With a deliberate effort, and with timely boosts from hands seen and unseen, my head rose above Ground Zero and the light was brighter than expected. Through new eyes I recognized this light as an incredible gift, which I am determined to share with others.